Ira Van Gieson

The correlation of sciences in the investigation of nervous and mental diseases

Ira Van Gieson

The correlation of sciences in the investigation of nervous and mental diseases

ISBN/EAN: 9783741171895

Manufactured in Europe, USA, Canada, Australia, Japa

Cover: Foto ©Lupo / pixelio.de

Manufactured and distributed by brebook publishing software
(www.brebook.com)

Ira Van Gieson

The correlation of sciences in the investigation of nervous and mental diseases

The ARCHIVES OF NEUROLOGY AND PSYCHOPATHOLOGY is published under the auspices of the New York State Hospitals and the Pathological Institute by permission of the State Commission in Lunacy. President, P. M. WISE, M. D.; Commissioners, GOODWIN BROWN and WILLIAM H. PARKHURST. : : : : : : : Edited for the State Hospitals by G. ALDER BLUMER, M. D., CHARLES W. PILGRIM, M. D., and SELDEN H. TALCOTT, M. D. : : : For the Pathological Institute by IRA VAN GIESON, M. D., BORIS SIDIS, PH. D., and HENDERSON B. DEADY, M. D. : : : : :

Vol. I . . . . . 1898 . . . . . Nos. 1–2.

Issued from the State Hospitals Press

at Utica, N. Y., December, 1898.

Pending two years devoted to the development of the organization and sphere of the scientific work of the State Hospitals and their centre of scientific research—the Pathological Institute of the New York State Hospitals—the STATE HOSPITALS BULLETIN has served as an organ for publication.

At present the plan and method of scientific investigation in the New York State Hospitals and Pathological Institute have become more defined, the lines of research of the several departments have become more completely organized, approaching more closely the original purpose of the foundation of a scientific centre of the New York State Hospitals—the plan of *correlation of sciences*, for the study of psychiatry.

This plan of scientific correlation in psychiatric research having during this period reached such a stage in its development as to unfold some definite results, it seems advisable to express the real character of our investigations, the outcome of this period of growth, in the title, more befitting the contents of the journal—ARCHIVES OF NEUROLOGY AND PSYCHOPATHOLOGY.

The ARCHIVES will contain studies on abnormal mental life and their neural concomitants, based on Psychology, Psychopathology, Experimental Physiology and Pathology, Cellular Biology, Pathological Anatomy, Comparative Neurology, Physiological Chemistry, Anthropolgy and Bacteriology.

EDITORS.

DECEMBER, 1898.

PLATE I

NEURON ENERGY AND ITS PSYCHOMOTOR MANIFESTATIONS.

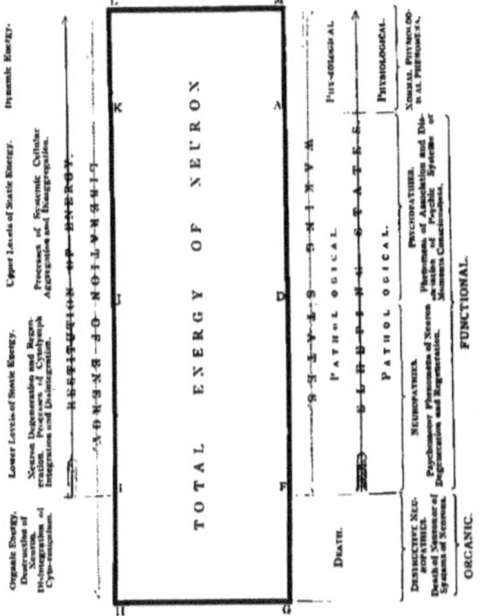

VOL. I 1898 No. 1

ARCHIVES

OF

NEUROLOGY AND PSYCHOPATHOLOGY

577.6

NEURON ENERGY AND ITS PSYCHOMOTOR MANIFESTATIONS.

(A PRELIMINARY COMMUNICATION).

IRA VAN GIESON, M. D. AND BORIS SIDIS, M. A., PH. D.

Director of the Pathological Institute of the New York State Hospitals.

Associate in Psychology and Psychopathology in the Pathological Institute of the New York State Hospitals.

We intend here to set forth in a concrete diagrammatic form a theory that attempts to correlate the various general manifestations of psychomotor life with more or less definite physiological processes depending on the expenditure or restitution of neuron energy.

If this theory were perhaps to open some new lines in the study of abnormal mental and neural manifestations, or if only to stimulate a reconsideration of some of the old problems, its publication is not inappropriate.

In the first plan (Plate I), the parallelogram G M L H represents the total energy of the neuron. This total energy of the neuron is divided into three phases, viz.: Dynamic, Static and Organic.

By *dynamic energy* of the neuron is meant that part of energy which the neuron as an individual organism can dispose of in its relations to other neurons forming complex functioning organizations.

The dynamic energy is represented by the upper portion of the parallelogram A M L K.

By *static energy* is designated that portion of energy that is used only for the life maintenance of the neuron, both in relation to other neurons and to its own inner molecular constitution. Static energy cannot be drawn upon by the neuron in its functioning activity with other neurons without bringing about a state of disintegration.

Static energy is indicated by the diagram A F K I.

By *organic energy* is meant that energy contained in the tissues of the dead neuron, not as yet decomposed into their inorganic constituents.

The reader should not be confused at the very outset in the consideration of these three phases of neuron energy, by supposing that they are different kinds of energy, in the sense of being distinct entities. This is not so. They merely represent three progressive phases or stages of the same process of neuron activity.

Liberation of neuron energy is correlative with *active* psychic or physical manifestations. Hence states of the nervous system corresponding to liberations of energy we have designated as *waking states*. *Restitution* of expended energy or *arrest* of liberation of neuron energy go hand in hand with *passive* conditions of the nervous system; hence states of restitution or arrest of energy we have termed collectively *sleeping states*.

In the first diagram, this correlation is followed out in the direction of the arrows. The downward arrow indicating successive levels of liberation of energy, corresponds to a similar downward arrow on the right hand side of the diagram, which indicates the course and progress of the waking states running parallel to the process of liberation of energy. The arrows on the left hand side of the diagram illustrate the physiological and pathological processes at work in the cycles of expenditure and restitution of energy, while the right hand side of the diagram indicates by its arrows the concomitant psychomotor manifestations—the waking and sleeping states.

The ascending arrow of restitution of energy corresponds to the ascending arrow on the right indicating the parallel psychomotor sleeping states. The descending arrows indicate physiological and pathological processes of liberation of energy and also their concomitant psychomotor waking states. Ascending and descending mean the rise and fall of the amount of energy, taking the upper level of dynamic energy as the starting point. Briefly stated, *descent* means *liberation* of energy with its concomitant psychomotor waking states. *Ascent* means *restitution* of energy with its parallel sleeping states.

The cycles in dynamic energy correspond to the physiological manifestations of the nervous system in the activity and rest of the individual in normal daily life. Concomitant with the expenditure of dynamic energy of the neurons, the individual passes through the active normal waking state, and hand in hand with the restitution of this expended dynamic energy, he passes through the sleeping state of normal daily life.

When, however, in the expenditure of energy, the border line or margin, A K, is crossed, dynamic energy is used up and static energy is drawn upon. The border line that separates the normal physiological from the abnormal or pathological psychomotor manifestations is stepped over.

Static energy may in its turn be divided into two phases according to the nature of the process of liberation of neuron energy. As long as the process of liberation of energy effects only a *dissociation* of systems of neurons the correlative psychomotor manifestations fall under the category of *psychopathies*. If, however, the process of liberation affects the neuron itself, bringing about a *disintegration* of its constituent parts compatible with restitution, the correlative psychomotor manifestations fall under the category of *neuropathies*. This process of disintegration, equivalent to cell degeneration in the patho-anatomical sense, may end in death, in the dissolution of the neuron itself.*

By *psychopathies*, then, we designate the pathological phenomena of *psychic disaggregation* correlative with the state or processes of dissociation within clusters or constellations of neurons, *the neuron itself remaining undamaged.*†

By *neuropathies*, we mean to indicate a group of psychophysical manifestations, running parallel to fluctuations of static energy and accompanied *by organic changes in the neuron.*

We may now turn to the larger and more complete schema.

The second chart (Plate II) is a further development of the first plan (Plate I). In it the pathological processes and their psychomotor concomitants are given in more or less provisional detail.

The *physiological* processes and corresponding psychomotor manifestations in the fluctuations of the *dynamic energy* hardly need, in the present communication, any further explanation, except possibly to indicate that

* Vide Sidis "Psychology of Suggestion." Ch. XXI, p. 214; Ch. XXIII, p. 234.

† The pathological phenomena of dissociation are discussed in full in "The Psychology of Suggestion."

dynamic energy is represented as expended and recruited by small or possibly infinitesmal differentials and increments. This is indicated by the parallel lines drawn across the rectangle representing dynamic energy, this energy falling or rising to different levels. Each of these increments is indicated by a fraction of the total energy, represented by the numerator e and the denominator n. The energy is assumed as drawn off, or recruited at any part of the whole rectangle by n^{ths} of the total amount.

Passing across the border line A K of the cyclic fluctuations corresponding to physiological metabolism constituted by the processes of catabolism and anabolism, fluctuations in the upper levels of the static energy of the neurons, are met with. Here we step over the catalytic threshold.

The physical processes occurring in the neuron, corresponding to these changes in the upper levels of the static energy, are no longer physiological, but pathological, and correspond to catalysis and synthesis.

Catalysis corresponds to liberation of the upper levels of static energy, and is accompanied by *retraction of aggregates of neurons*, bringing about the phenomena of psychophysiological dissociation. Restitution of the energy expended in the catalytic process is accompanied by *expansion* or *synthesis* of the neurons which are again able to transmit or receive impulses in the particular aggregate to which they belong.* An arrest or halt after the expenditure of energy in these upper static levels, corresponds again to a state of retraction of the neuron or catalysis.†

On the right hand side of the diagram, concomitant

* For further details see Sidis "Psychology of Suggestion," Chap. XXI, XXIII.

† Apathy's "anastamosis" theory may hold true of the nervous system of the invertebrates, but not of the cerebro-spinal system and certainly not of the association areas. This topic will form the subject of a separate work.

with the processes of catalysis or synthesis of the neuron, we find corresponding pathological states of psychic dis-aggregation and aggregation: *psychopathic waking states* or states of mental dissociation going hand in hand with *catalysis*, and *psychopathic sleeping states* with the process of *synthesis*.

In the second column, on the right hand side of the diagram, a general outline is given of the detailed manifestations of the psychopathic waking states. These are given in the sequence in which they occur, as far as we can determine in the present writing, according to the progression of the catalytic process passing from the very highest constellations of neurons which the nervous system possesses, down through lower and lower associations and finally to groups of neurons.*

In the third column to the right of the central rectangle in the diagram are given some of the specific manifestations of the neuron associations during the psychopathic sleeping state, when the upper levels of static energy have reached the maximum of their expenditure, and ascend toward the normal physiological level by the process of restitution of energy.

These cycles in the rise or fall of energy are always indicated by the direction of the smaller arrows on either side of the central rectangle, representing the total energy of the neuron.

Psychopathic manifestations correspond to the processes of catalysis and synthesis of the neurons, or to an arrest in the liberation of energy after catalysis has progressed to a certain degree.

Passing now beyond the catalytic margin in the expenditure of static energy of the neuron, we may consider

* Vide Sidis "Psychology of Suggestion," Chap. XX and XXI.

the further expenditure of static energy. Here we step over the cytolytic threshold. The pathological process corresponding to expenditure of the levels of static energy beneath the cytolytic threshold is termed *cytolysis* of the neuron, which means cell-resolution. At this point organic and structural changes are found in the neuron, more particularly in the character of the cytolymph.* We have here the *initial stages of the process of neuron degeneration*, and the term cytolysis indicates such phases of parenchymatous degeneration of the neurons which may lead either to restitution or destruction. Cytolysis, therefore, embraces the phases of organic degeneration of the neurons up to, but not beyond the border line of destruction in the progression of this degeneration.

The regeneration of these degenerative changes in the cell, not over-stepping the limits of destructive alterations in the neuron, is termed *cytothesis*. It is the reverse of cytolysis.

Corresponding again to the pathological processes of cytolysis and cytothesis, going hand in hand with fluctuations in the lower levels of static energy, are the concomitant *neuropathic* waking and sleeping states with their psychomotor manifestations.

Broadly speaking, psychopathies run parallel to the phenomena of retraction and expansion of aggregates of neurons, while neuropathies are concomitant with actual degeneration of the neuron, especially of its cytolymph.

The expenditure of organic energy is accompanied with cell-destruction or *cytoclasis*.† Cytoclasis is the destructive outcome of degeneration of the neurons—parenchymatous degeneration of the nervous system, acute or chronic.

* For further details of these processes see van Gieson "The Toxic Basis of Neural Diseases," begun in a previous issue of the STATE HOSPITALS BULLETIN.

† Vide van Gieson, "Toxic Basis of Neural Diseases."

There can be neither waking nor sleeping states below the cytolytic margin, as the neuron is dead.*

In setting down the specific symptomatic expressions of the several psychopathic and neuropathic sleeping and waking states, it is impossible, in many instances, to draw sharp lines of division between the two sets. They are necessarily put down in a general way, and more or less provisionally as an attempt to analyze psychomotor phenomena manifested in abnormal nervous and mental life on a tangible basis of fluctuations of neuron energy.

The difficulty of sharply defining abnormal waking and sleeping states of the nervous system lies in the fact that in the same individual one part of the nervous system is in the process of restitution and is in a sleeping state, while another portion is in the process of expending energy and is in a waking state.

The reader should also be guarded from receiving the impression that sleeping stadia of the nervous system necessarily go hand in hand with a progressive upward rise of the process of energy restitution. It is always to be remembered that the downward process in the liberation of energy is not necessarily followed by the opposite cycle of restitution of energy. The process may halt, or, strictly speaking, *oscillate*, at some particular level, as at B, C, or D, (in the central rectangle) when a sleeping state is liable to predominate, because from the very nature of pathological metabolism the ascending processes are slower in their course than the descending processes. The liberation process may then, without rising, descend to a still deeper level, as at E. It may then rise to C, and fall back to D, and so on through an almost indefinite

* Vide Sidis "Psychology of Suggestion," pp. 214, 232.

series of halts,—upward and downward fluctuations. This ought to make clear our conception of the progression of the sleeping and waking states. Thus, the pathological process and symptoms concurrent with the expenditure of successive levels of static energy may descend and continually go down deeper into the psychopathic and neuropathic realms of psychomotor manifestations. Finally, the descent may be so great that the liberation of energy corresponds to the destruction of the nerve cell, and the disease becomes permanent. The earliest manifestations of general paresis, for instance, are those corresponding to the liberations or restitutions of the uppermost levels of static energy, but finally the process of liberation reaches such a depth that the disease becomes destructive. *Psychopathies may therefore become neuropathies, and neuropathies may in their turn progress to the cytoclastic type and result in an absolute and irrevocable loss of function of the neuron.**

The fluctuations of energy again may be such as to take a pronounced alternating or cyclical type, and herein, we believe, is a rational explanation of the circular insanities. *The active periods of the circular insanities belong to waking states, and the passive periods are sleeping states of the nervous system.* This holds true not only of psychopathic, but also of neuropathic circular states—states of alternating delirium and coma such as are found in the acute general somatic diseases that involve the nervous system. The active delirium is placed on the side of the vertical line to be included in the neuropathic waking states, and the passive or comatose alternation of the neuropathic psychic manifestations is set down among the neuropathic sleeping states.

* Vide Sidis "Psychology of Suggestion," Chap. XXIII, pp. 215, 232.

It should be remembered that the psychopathic cyclic insanities may not at all remain fixed where they begin in the psychopathic realm, they may descend into the neuropathic domain. In the consideration of this second chart in general, it is always to be held in mind that the order in which these phenomena are set down in the psychopathic and neuropathic states is an order both serial and progressive and no particular set of symptoms is to be considered as fixed in this scale, except as to its course and origin. Thus psychopathic may descend into neuropathic waking states and these again into the domain of destruction of the nerve cell. On the other hand, neuropathic sleeping states may rise to the level of psychopathic sleeping states. Cytoclastic states, however, cannot rise, there can be no restitution because the neuron is destroyed. If *any recovery from cytoclasis does occur, it is because of a compensatory action of other neurons and an education on the part of new neurons to assume the functions lost by their destroyed associates.*

It must be distinctly understood, that while the parenchymatous degeneration associated with these several pathological processes begins as a cytolytic lesion, compatible with restitution and recovery of the neuron, it may pass on to the destructive state. No one can say, in treating of these nervous diseases generically, whether they may become cytoclastic or remain cytolytic and susceptible of recovery. The determination of such a question must be sought out in the special conditions of each particular case.

Furthermore, the important fact must be kept clearly in mind that various groups and systems of neurons may reach different degrees of disaggregation and degeneration, may be simultaneously in different stages of the one continuous descending pathological process of energy liberation. A community, cluster or constellation of neuron aggregates, *A*, may be in the upper levels of the psychopathic state; another, *B*, in the deeper levels of the same state; *C* and *D* in different levels of the neuropathic state, while *E* and *F* may have descended to the levels of cytoclasis. Such a complexity of phenomena is well illustrated in general paresis. Thus the fact that various systems of neurons are often in different stages of disaggregation or degeneration frequently gives rise to a mixed and complex symptomatology, the malady presenting symptoms (psychomotor manifestations) belonging to different stages in the descending pathological process. The disease, however, may still be characterized as *psychopathic*, if *most* of the neuron aggregates are in the psychopathic state; it may be designated *neuropathic*, if *most* of the neuron aggregates are in the neuropathic state; it may be termed *cytoclastic*, if *most* of the neuron aggregates involved in the process, have reached the destructive stage of cell degeneration. The symptomatology of psychomotor manifestations may thus vary endlessly, like the figures in the kaleidoscope. The *symptomatic side of disease is a function of* LOCATION, NUMBER *and* DEGREE. *It depends on the location and number of neuron aggregates involved and on the stage or degree of the descending pathological process.*

We must be clear in reference to some other points.

First, neuron energy may be liberated even in the dynamic and static levels not as psychomotor manifestations, but as heat, electricity, etc.

Secondly, the dissipation of *organic* energy of the neuron takes the form of chemical energy in the dissolution of the bodies composing the cyto-reticulum or in giving rise to heat or electric currents. These two latter forms of energy are of no special interest in connection with psychomotor manifestations, they fall outside the domain of *functional* energy of the neuron, the subject matter of this communication. This liberation of non-nervous energy from destruction of the cyto-reticulum is the reason of the prolongation of the descending arrow beyond the cytolytic margin.

Thirdly, we do not believe that a sleeping state of the nervous system can occur without an antecedent waking state. The patient may not come under observation, during this antecedent waking state, and as a matter of fact rarely does in those psychopathic waking stages where the attack is acute and the liberation process is of a very short duration. The active waking state corresponding to liberation of energy, preceding what is supposed to be the primary depressed state, may be sudden, fleeting, unobtrusive, but it must exist. *An individual cannot be precipitated into a sleeping state without having gone through an antecedent active or waking state.*

To complete this chart a whole domain of psychomotor manifestations is requisite, namely, that corresponding to the fluctuations of neuron energy, containing the mixed phenomena of simultaneous waking and sleeping states. These states, as well as many other conditions, require a careful experimental investigation from the standpoint of our theory.

Finally, it should be noted that the division lines, such as lie between the cycles of physiological and the subdivisions of the cycles of pathological metabolism, are rather relative. One process directly and continuously passes over into the other; thus catalysis is the forerunner of cytolysis, and cytolysis may become the forerunner of cytoclasis. *All of them, however, are stages in the one continuous process of liberation of neuron energy.**

* Vide Sidis "Psychology of Suggestion," pp. 214, 215, 232.

The various nervous and mental diseases are generally considered as separate things. Each disease is assumed as standing by itself, an independent clinical entity, an "Anundfürsichsein." This view is metaphysical, although it would seem that nothing is so far removed from metaphysics as medical science. Now, as a matter of fact, *diseases are not entities*, *but processes. Particular sets of symptoms characterizing different clinical pictures of nervous and mental diseases form stages in the one continuous process of liberation of neuron energy of the specially affected neuron aggregates.*

This one continuous process of liberation of neuron energy may cover the life of a single individual or may extend over the life-history of many generations. The continuous descending pathological process may spread out in time and space, may extend over a long duration of time and embrace a great number of individuals. The tide of neuron energy may ebb away gradually, leaving each succeeding generation on a lower stage and deeper level in the continuous process of neuron disaggregation and degeneration, thus giving rise to the different stages and manifestations of *congenital degeneracy*. Many of the so-called degeneracies and the congenital diseases of the nervous system arise, we believe, in this way.

In the higher parts of the nervous system pathological processes begin in catalysis, on further descent pass into cytolysis, and if continued further terminate into cytoclasis. In these regions *catalysis*, *cytolysis*, *cytoclasis*, *are the three progressive descending stages in the complete cycle of pathological processes*. In the lower and lowermost neural segments, however, pathological processes may lack catalysis and begin in cytolysis.

The processes of liberation and restitution of neuron

energy may be symbolically represented in the following formulæ:

Let D represent the physiological or dynamic energy of the neuron, S its static, and R its organic energy, then $D+S+R=E$, or total energy of neuron; that is

$$D+S+R=E \quad (1).$$

Let $\frac{e}{n}$ be the differential (see Plate II, rectangle K A M L) liberated by each successive or progressive increment of stimulus, then a progressive series arises, the summation of which will be equal to D, or

$$D-(\tfrac{e}{n}+\tfrac{e}{n}+\tfrac{e}{n}+\tfrac{e}{n}+\tfrac{e}{n}+\ldots.\tfrac{e}{n}+\tfrac{e}{n})=0 \quad (2)$$

This represents a progressive descending series in the course of neuron activity of the physiological waking state corresponding to the process of catabolism. If we subtract D or the sum of the descending progressive series from E, or total energy, we have static and organic energies or

$$E-(\tfrac{e}{n}+\tfrac{e}{n}+\tfrac{e}{n}+\tfrac{e}{n}+\tfrac{e}{n}+\ldots\ldots.\tfrac{e}{n}+\tfrac{e}{n})=S+R \quad (3)$$

Having descended and reached S, the process of liberation may continue, but at this point it passes into the regions of *pathological waking states.* The process of liberation continues in the same way by $\frac{e}{n}$ decrements.

Now S may be divided into two separate but continuous series representing two stages of the pathological waking state in the progressively descending scale of liberation of neuron energy. The first series corresponds to catalysis, the second to cytolysis.

The process of liberation of organic energy of the neuron R corresponds to cytoclasis.

If the static energy liberated by catalysis be designated by C, the energy liberated by cytolysis by C_1, and the organic energy set free by cytoclasis by C_2, then we have the following formulæ:

$$C - \left(\tfrac{e}{n}+\tfrac{e}{n}+\tfrac{e}{n}+\tfrac{e}{n}+\ldots\ldots\tfrac{e}{n}+\tfrac{e}{n}\right)=0 \quad (4) \text{ Catalytic margin.}$$

$$C_1 - \left(\tfrac{e}{n}+\tfrac{e}{n}+\tfrac{e}{n}+\tfrac{e}{n}+\ldots\ldots\tfrac{e}{n}+\tfrac{e}{n}\right)=0 \quad (5) \text{ Cytolytic margin.}$$

$$C_2 - \left(\tfrac{e}{n}+\tfrac{e}{n}+\tfrac{e}{n}+\tfrac{e}{n}+\ldots\ldots\tfrac{e}{n}+\tfrac{e}{n}\right)=0 \quad (6) \text{ Cytoclastic terminus.}$$

These formulæ express respectively the limits of liberation of energy of the three descending pathological processes.

Adding equations (4), (5), (6) together, we have:

$$(C+C_1+C_2)-\left[\left(\tfrac{e}{n}+\tfrac{e}{n}+\tfrac{e}{n}+\ldots\ldots\tfrac{e}{n}+\tfrac{e}{n}\right)+\left(\tfrac{e}{n}+\tfrac{e}{n}+\tfrac{e}{n}+\ldots\ldots\tfrac{e}{n}+\tfrac{e}{n}\right)+\left(\tfrac{e}{n}+\tfrac{e}{n}+\tfrac{e}{n}+\ldots\ldots\tfrac{e}{n}+\tfrac{e}{n}\right)\right]=0 \quad (7)$$

With the final decrement of equation (5) we reach the functional zero point or cytolytic margin and with the final term of equation (6) we reach the absolute zero point, the terminus of liberation of energy. The cytolytic margin indicates the end of the expenditure of *nervous* or *functional* energy; the cytoclastic terminus marks the close of the residual or *non-nervous* energy of the neuron. The lowest limit in the descending process of energy dissipation is reached at the cytoclastic terminus of the total cell energy. This terminus may be represented in the following formulæ:

$$E-D-S-R=E-D-(C+C_1+C_2)=0 \quad (8) \text{ or,}$$

$$E-\left[\left(\tfrac{e}{n}+\tfrac{e}{n}+\tfrac{e}{n}+\ldots\ldots\tfrac{e}{n}+\tfrac{e}{n}\right)+\left(\tfrac{e}{n}+\tfrac{e}{n}+\ldots\ldots\tfrac{e}{n}+\tfrac{e}{n}\right)+\left(\tfrac{e}{n}+\tfrac{e}{n}+\tfrac{e}{n}\ldots\tfrac{e}{n}+\tfrac{e}{n}\right)+\left(\tfrac{e}{n}+\tfrac{e}{n}+\tfrac{e}{n}\ldots+\tfrac{e}{n}+\tfrac{e}{n}\right)\right]=0 \quad (9)$$

Recapitulating the whole process of the continuous progressive *descending* series of liberation of nervous cell energy from the *minimum* to the *maximum* limit, we have the following formula:

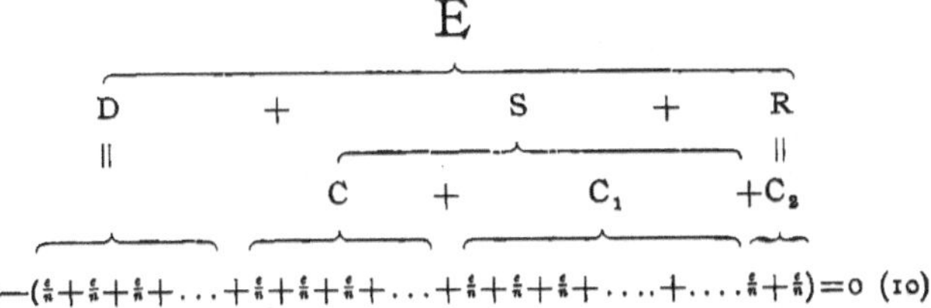

$$E-\left(\frac{e}{n}+\frac{e}{n}+\frac{e}{n}+\ldots+\frac{e}{n}+\frac{e}{n}+\frac{e}{n}+\ldots+\frac{e}{n}+\frac{e}{n}+\frac{e}{n}+\ldots\ldots+\ldots\ldots\frac{e}{n}+\frac{e}{n}\right)=0 \quad (10)$$

Each term in the descending series of liberation of functional or nervous energy manifests itself as a waking state, physiological, *i.e.*, catabolic; or pathological, *i.e.*, catalytic and cytolytic, according to the depth of the descent.

Having formulated the descending series of liberation of nerve-cell energy, we turn now to the formulation of the process of restitution of energy which takes place in an *ascending* series.

If in the equation (2) the number of terms be M, the summation of them will give $M\frac{e}{n}$, then in the complete integration of the ascending series concomitant with the anabolic physiological sleeping state we have:

$$D=M\frac{e}{n} \quad (11)$$

In a similar way we may integrate the pathological series in the ascending scale of restitution, namely, equations (4) and (5). The summation of equation (4) which we may suppose as having M_1 terms in the ascending series of the synthetic sleeping state will give us the following formula:

$$C=M_1\frac{e}{n} \quad (12)$$

The summation of equation (5) which we may suppose

as having M_2 terms in the ascending series of the cytothetic sleeping state will give the following formula:

$$C_1 = M_2 \tfrac{e}{n} \quad (13)$$

The series of cytoclasis cannot be integrated as restitution, from the very nature of the destructive character of the cytoclastic process, is impossible.

Thus far we have dealt with *complete* cycles in the descending scale of liberation of energy concomitant with waking states and the ascending scale of restitution concomitant with sleeping states. Each cycle, however, may be incomplete, may stop and oscillate at any point in the scale of the series. Thus the ascending process of integration or restitution of energy may be only $\tfrac{e}{n}$, or $2\tfrac{e}{n}$, or $3\tfrac{e}{n}, \ldots\ldots\ldots$ or $(M-1)\tfrac{e}{n}$ of the expended nervous energy. The restitution of these increments may be characterized as *positive* and indicated by (+).

The same holds true in the case of the process of loss or liberation of neuron energy, it may descend and reach any point in the descending series. The dynamic energy D, for instance, may lose the decrement, $\tfrac{e}{n}$, or decrements $2\tfrac{e}{n}$, $3\tfrac{e}{n} \ldots\ldots\ldots (M-1)\tfrac{e}{n}$, $M\tfrac{e}{n}$, and become $D-\tfrac{e}{n}$, $D-2\tfrac{e}{n}$, $D-3\tfrac{e}{n} \ldots\ldots\ldots D-(M-1)\tfrac{e}{n}$, $D-M\tfrac{e}{n}$. These losses or decrements of liberation of energy may be characterized as *negative* and indicated by (−).

Since the descending process of liberation of cell energy is divided into four stages, one merging into the other, namely, the catabolic, the catalytic, the cytolytic and the cytoclastic, and since the reverse series of the ascending process is divided into three stages, one passing into the other, namely, the cytothetic, the synthetic and the anabolic, it would be well to co-ordinate these processes and their stages and represent them by the following comprehensive formula:

WAKING STATES.

(14)

Physiological. — Liberation of Dynamic Energy.

Catabolism.	*Anabolism.*
D.................	$M\frac{e}{n}$
$D-\frac{e}{n}$...............	$(M-1)\frac{e}{n}$
$D-2\frac{e}{n}$..............	$(M-2)\frac{e}{n}$
$D-3\frac{e}{n}$..............	$(M-3)\frac{e}{n}$
$D-4\frac{e}{n}$..............	$(M-4)\frac{e}{n}$
....	....
....	....
....	....
$D-(M-1)\frac{e}{n}$..........	$\frac{e}{n}$
$D-M\frac{e}{n}$............	o

Restitution of Dynamic Energy. — Physiological.

(15)

Psychopathic. — Liberation of Upper Levels of Static Energy.

Catalysis.	*Synthesis.*
C.................	$M_1\frac{e}{n}$
$C-\frac{e}{n}$...............	$(M_1-1)\frac{e}{n}$
$C-2\frac{e}{n}$..............	$(M_1-2)\frac{e}{n}$
$C-3\frac{e}{n}$..............	$(M_1-3)\frac{e}{n}$
$C-4\frac{e}{n}$..............	$(M_1-4)\frac{e}{n}$
....	....
....	....
....	....
$C-(M_1-1)\frac{e}{n}$.........	$\frac{e}{n}$
$C-M_1\frac{e}{n}$...........	o

Restitution of Upper Levels of Static Energy. — Psychopathic.

(16)

Neuropathic. — Liberation of Lower Levels of Static Energy.

Cytolysis.	*Cytothesis.*
C_1..................	$M_2\frac{e}{n}$
$C_1-\frac{e}{n}$...............	$(M_2-1)\frac{e}{n}$
$C_1-2\frac{e}{n}$..............	$(M_2-2)\frac{e}{n}$
$C_1-3\frac{e}{n}$..............	$(M_2-3)\frac{e}{n}$
$C_1-4\frac{e}{n}$..............	$(M_2-4)\frac{e}{n}$
....	....
....	....
....	....
$C_1-(M_2-1\frac{e}{n})$........	$\frac{e}{n}$
$C_1-M_2\frac{e}{n}$	o

Restitution of Lower Levels of Static Energy. — Neuropathic.

SLEEPING STATES.

Cytolytic Margin. (Exhaustion of Cyto-lymph).

Liberation of Non-Nervous Energy—Heat, Chemical Energy.

Cytoclasis.

C_2

$C_2-\frac{e}{n}$

$C_2-2\frac{e}{n}$

$C_2-3\frac{e}{n}$

$C_2-4\frac{e}{n}$

....

....

Cytoclastic Terminus of Neuron Energy.

(Destruction of Cyto-reticulum).

Formulæ (14), (15) and (16) illustrate the phases of seeming arrests, but really of oscillations in the progression of the processes of liberation or restitution of energy. In catalysis, for instance, liberation of energy may oscillate at the level, $C-\frac{e}{n}$, when a sleeping state may predominate. The catalytic process may then descend to a lower stage of the series, $C-4\frac{e}{n}$, and during the descent there is a waking state. If an oscillation occurs at the level, $C-4\frac{e}{n}$, a sleeping state again preponderates. Certain cases of cyclical insanity manifesting alternations of waking and sleeping states with slight or no restitution of energy may serve as a case in point. The process of liberation of energy has slipped from one level to a deeper one, thence to a still deeper level, oscillating for a period at each of these levels. In the same way, in formula (15), in the right hand column of series, corresponding to the synthetic process, we may have a similar symbolical illustration of oscillatory periods in the restitution of energy.

The upper levels of static energy in any particular individual may be reduced to the catalytic margin, the process of disintegration may become arrested at this point and the reverse process of synthesis may begin; the process of restitution of energy may rise by $\frac{e}{n}$ths. The recuperation of the energy corresponding to synthesis may rise say to $(M_1-4)\frac{e}{n}$ (formula 15, right hand column); after oscillating there a while it may rise to a higher level of the series such as $(M_1-1)\frac{e}{n}$, and so on until all the upper levels of static energy expressed by the final member of the ascending series, $M_1\frac{e}{n}$, are recovered. The individual has recovered all the upper levels of his static energy and is on the way to become normal; he is about to step across the border line into the realm of the normal physiological sleeping state.

We may conclude this brief preliminary communication with a few laws relating to the metabolic processes of neuron activity:

(I)—*Catalysis stands in direct and synthesis in inverse ratio to the number of disaggregated neuron associations.*

(II)—All other conditions remaining the same, *the instability of a cell aggregate is proportionate to the* number *and* complexity *of its associative functioning groups.**

(III)—*The stability of a neuron aggregate is proportionate to the* frequency *and* duration *of its associative activity.*†

(IV)—*The instability of a neuron aggregate is proportionate to the* frequency *and* duration *of the* interruptions *in its functioning activity.*‡

(V)—*The mass of formed metaplasm granules*‖ *stands in direct ratio to the intensity of cytolysis and in inverse ratio to the progress of cytothesis.*

* See Sidis, Psychology of Suggestion, p. 212.

† Ibid, p. 210.

‡ For further details, particularly in relation to the many forms of psychopathies, see the second part of The Psychology of Suggestion, especially Chapters XX, XXI, XXII, XXIII.

‖ "Metaplasm granules" is a term given by one of us, in order to be more explicit about the significance of the commonly called pigment granules of the ganglion cell. Metaplasm granules are the lifeless particles in the neuron, excreted from it; they are waste products attending the liberation of energy, especially pathological liberations, from the cytolymph; hence we think that the volume of these metaplasm granules is a measure of the declining capacity of the cytolymph to elaborate and liberate neuron energy. Vide van Gieson, "Toxic Basis of Neural Diseases."

TOTAL ENERGY OF NEURON.

DYNAMIC. — CYCLE OF PHYSIOLOGICAL METABOLISM.

CATABOLISM (OF THE NEURON)
Liberation of dynamic energy of the neuron.

ANABOLISM (OF THE NEURON)
Integration—Restitution of liberated dynamic energy.

CATABOLIC MARGIN. (Limit of Catabolic Process.)
CATALYTIC THRESHOLD.

STATIC. — CYCLES OF PATHOLOGICAL METABOLISM.

DISAGGREGATION AND AGGREGATION OF NEURONS.

DENDRITIC RETRACTION. = NEURON CATALYSIS.
Liberation of static energy.

DENDRITIC EXPANSION. = NEURON SYNTHESIS
Integration of static energy liberated by the catalytic process.

CATALYTIC MARGIN. (Limit of Catalytic Process.)
CYTOLYTIC THRESHOLD.

CELL RESOLUTION AND RESTITUTION.

CELL RESOLUTION. = NEURON CYTOLYSIS
Further progressive liberation of static energy beyond catalysis.

CELL RESTITUTION. = NEURON CYTOTHESIS
Integration of static energy liberated by the cytolytic process.

CYTOLYTIC MARGIN. (Limit of Cytolytic Process.)
CYTOCLASTIC THRESHOLD.

ORGANIC. — Cell Destruction.

CELL DESTRUCTION. = CYTOCLASIS (OF THE NEURON)
Progressive liberation of organic energy.

* See Sidis "Psychology of Suggestion," Part II, Chapters XX, XXI, XXII, XXIII.

LIBERATION OF ENERGY OF THE NEURON.

RESTITUTION OF ENERGY OF THE NEURON.

WAKING STATES. — SLEEPING STATES.

PSYCHOMOTOR MANIFESTATIONS (SYMPTOMATOLOGY).

NORMAL. — ABNORMAL: PSYCHOPATHIES. NEUROPATHIES.

PHYSIOLOGICAL WAKING STATES. — Waking Phase of Daily Normal Life.

PHYSIOLOGICAL SLEEPING STATES. — Sleeping States of Normal Daily Life. Dream States.

PHYSIOLOGICAL MARGIN. (Limit of Sense of Fatigue.)
PSYCHOPATHIC THRESHOLD.

PSYCHOPATHIC WAKING STATES.

PSYCHOPATHIC SLEEPING STATES.

PSYCHOPATHIC MARGIN.
NEUROPATHIC THRESHOLD.

NEUROPATHIC WAKING STATES.

NEUROPATHIC SLEEPING STATES.

NEUROPATHIC MARGIN.

DEATH OF NEURON.

THE CORRELATION OF SCIENCES IN THE INVESTIGATION OF NERVOUS AND MENTAL DISEASES.*

IRA VAN GIESON, M. D.,
Director of the Pathological Institute of the New York State Hospitals.

"No one can have a firm grasp of any science if, by confining himself to it, he shuts out the light of analogy, and deprives himself of that peculiar aid which is derived from a commanding survey of the co-ordination and interdependence of things and of the relation they bear to each other. He may, no doubt, work at the details of his subject; he may be useful in adding to its facts; he will never be able to enlarge its philosophy. For, the philosophy of every department depends on its connection with other departments, and must therefore be sought at their points of contact. It must be looked for in the place where they touch and coalesce; it lies not in the centre of each science, but on the confines and margin."—*Buckle's Essay on Mill.*

PART I.

PSYCHIATRY, ITS GROWTH AND METHODS.

CHAPTER I.

THE HISTORY OF PSYCHIATRY.

The history of the insane has been written again and again, and is familiar to all who deal with this unfortunate and dependent class; still a glance at this growth and progress of psychiatric work gives such graphic and incontestible evidence of the absolute dependence of the progress of the treatment of the insane upon science,

* This paper is in substance a report presenting the purpose of the Pathological Institute of the New York State Hospitals to the State Commission in Lunacy for transmission to the legislature. From its nature it had to be written in an untechnical form. As this paper not only endeavors to forecast the work of the State Hospitals and the Institute but also covers the scope of their official publications, it may not be inappropriate to publish this text in the ARCHIVES, with such modifications as have been found indispensable.

that I may ask for indulgence in once more tracing the outlines of this chronicle.

In the early Egyptian, Babylonian, Assyrian and Biblical periods, the whole subject of insanity was entirely wrapt up in the grossest superstition and relegated to the influence of good or evil spirits. The ancient Egyptian understood well enough what every other civilized nation has found out by observation, namely, the enormously destructive effects of alcohol upon the human brain. An ancient papyrus exhorting a drunkard to forsake the tavern, states "that if beer gets into a man, it overcomes the mind."

Biblical illustrations of insanity are too familiar to need mention. The insanity of Saul, Nebuchadnezzar, and the feigned insanity of King David are household knowledge. The healing of the lunatic in the New Testament describes the classical symptoms of epilepsy, and the deportment of the swine after being pervaded by the devils or unclean spirits, cast out of the Gergesene madman, gives a graphic illustration of the objective character and individuality of demoniacal possession in insanity.

A glance at the status of insanity among the Greeks is very interesting. The Hellenic world regarded insanity as a visitation of the Gods. This was natural and in harmony with the elaborate character of their mythology. Homer tells how the anger of the Gods reduced Bellerophon to melancholia and Sophocles describes the furious and destructive mania of Ajax terminating in melancholia. Euripides gives such a fine description of the cardinal symptoms of an attack of homicidal fury with epilepsy that it might well pass as the description of a well informed modern psychiatrist.

The first protest against the superstition and ignorance

in which this subject was enveloped is found in the writings of Hippocrates. Hippocrates was wonderfully in advance of his times. Here was a physician and a man of scientific knowledge, practising in the fifth century before Christ,.yet his bold, self-reliant opposition to superstition and ignorance always kindles new admiration. He wastes no words in battering down the makeshift of ascribing misunderstood things to the Divinity, the invariable refuge of the ignorant.

In speaking of epilepsy the "Sacred Disease," he says: "The sacred disease appears to me no wise more Divine nor more sacred than other diseases; but has a natural cause from which it originates like other affections. Men regard its nature and cause as Divine from ignorance and wonder, because it is not at all like other diseases." He also brings out the inconsistency of singling out epilepsy as the sacred disease since so many kindred affections of the brain of equally mysterious origin ought equally well be called Divine or sacred diseases. He remarks again: "They who first referred this disease to the gods appear to me to have been just such persons as the conjurors, purificators, mountebanks and charlatans now are. * * * Such persons, then, using the Divinity as a pretext, and screen for their own inability to afford any assistance, have given out that the disease is sacred, adding suitable reasons for the opinion, and they have instituted a mode of treatment which is safe for themselves, namely, by applying purifications and incantations and enforcing abstinence from baths and many articles of food, which are unwholesome to men in disease. * * * *This disease is formed from those things which enter into and go out of the body* and it is not more difficult to understand and cure than the others, neither is it more Divine than other diseases.

* * * "Men ought to know that from nothing else but the brain (the soul and with it physic manifestations was located in the stomach by one eminent physician of the middle ages) come joy, despondency and lamentation * * * and by the same organ we become *mad* and *delirious*." These are fine, blunt, common sense words from a scientific man, and it is a pity that they remained unheeded for two thousand years.

Hippocrates' hint as to the causal agency of epilepsy in the italicised sentence is particularly interesting, for even to-day we have only begun to search out whether epileptic attacks may not be due to the action on the brain of some poison which escapes from the intestines into the blood in course of disordered digestion. Hippocrates clearly points out too that disease of the brain is accountable for insanity. Besides this he even classified insanity with such good sense into manias, melancholias and dementia, that in 90 per cent of the cases at the present day the self-same classification is used.

Furthermore he believed that diseases of the brain were caused by "bad humors." And if the term "bad humors" be translated as poisons or toxic agents it is the scientific language which we have just begun to employ in explaining the cause of many forms of insanity.

This remarkable man went even further. He proposed *treatment* and *cure* of the insane, by ridding and purging the body of these brain disturbing humors.

The next champion of enlightenment with regard to the insane, appears in Asclepiades, about 100 B. C. He protested against poisoning patients with opium and hyoscyamus, but tried to "induce sleep by gentle friction." He would not tolerate venesection, nor dark cells, but brought his patients out into the light and gave them an efficient diet which although somewhat abstemious was systematic and regular.

The renowned Celsus living somewhat later is rather disappointing in his treatment of the insane, for what good there was in his moral treatment, was overbalanced by the abuse of the insane, making them "capitulate," by starving, binding in chains and in beating them. His influence in subsequent periods was also pernicious, for as Tuke remarks: "It is melancholy to reflect that many centuries afterwards, all that was bad in his system was faithfully copied and even intensified, while what was good (the music, the sports, and the excitement of cheerful hopes) was overlooked; as was also the employment of friction—in other words, massage and regular exercise after food."

Of all names illustrious in the rescue of the insane from Hippocrates down to the times of men of Pinel's stamp, that of Caelius Aurelianus stands alone and unrivalled. The isolated brilliancy of this man is due to scientific knowledge and the attributes of courage of convictions, common sense and humanity. Moreover, all this in the man was happily joined with a faculty of practical application in the salvation of the insane. I can do no better than to quote from Dr. Tuke as to what this man accomplished:

"He had no patience with those who reduced a violent patient to obedience by flagellation which he speaks of as applied to the face and head, and so causing swellings and sores. He recognized the mental pain from which the unfortunate would suffer on returning to consciousness. He placed the maniac in a room, moderately light and warm and excluded everything of an exciting character. His bed was to be firm, properly fixed to the floor, and situated so that the patient would not be disturbed by seeing persons enter the room. Straw, soft and well beaten, but not broken, was to be used for the bed, and if the patient tried to injure himself, he was to be padded on the neck and chest with soft wool."

"Minute and praiseworthy were the rules laid down by the enlightened physician, as to the duties of *attendants* and it would not disgrace, says Dr. Tuke, the corresponding regulations in the hand-book prepared by the Scotch branch of the Medico-Psychological Association. Thus they were to beware of appearing to confirm the patient's delusions and so deepen his malady. They were to take care not to exasperate him by needless opposition and they were to endeavor to correct his delusions at one time by indulging condescension and at another by insinuations. Fomentations by means of warm sponges were to be applied over the eyelids in order to relax them, and at the same time to exert a beneficial influence on the membranes of the brain."

"Restlessness and sleeplessness were to be relieved by carrying the patient about on a litter. During convalescence theatrical entertainments were to be given. * * .* Riding, walking and the exertion of the voice were recommended. For the poorer patients, *farming* was to be encouraged if they were agriculturists, while if sailors they were to be allowed to go on the water. He denounced the abstinence which Celsus had extolled and asserted that a low diet was more calculated to cause than to cure madness. Further he protested in the strongest manner against putting patients in chains and trusted to the care and control exercised by attendants. He speaks against the practice pursued by some of making patients intoxicated, inasmuch as insanity was often caused by drink. He was opposed to venesection (but not to cupping) and to reducing the strength of the patient by the administration of hellebore and aloes, on the contrary, he favored soothing and invigorating the patient by emollient or astringent application."

The work of this man does not need much comment. It speaks for itself. He is the Pinel of ancient times—a firm indomitable humane apostle of science, striking off the manacles of the insane, neglecting the twaddle of superstition and instituting measures for treatment and cure. In short, he took the insane out of the dungeons, bedlams and infernos, and placed them in hospitals, where they belong like other human beings afflicted with diseases of other organs than the brain. All this we in the light of modern times have only brought into general use within the last twenty or fifty years. The man was some seventeen hundred years in advance of his times.

Thus we find that even in ancient times science rescued the insane from the hades of superstition and reached its climax in caring for and treating them in the enlightened hospital of Aurelianus, the forerunner of the great modern hospitals of the present day in our own State. This took some four hundred years from the times of Hippocrates to Aurelianus (first century A. D.) The remarkable thing in this epoch of progress in psychiatry, is the fact that it was accomplished by three or four great leading men not even operating consecutively much less collectively, and in the face of a mythology which firmly pervaded almost all walks of life. When a man like Hippocrates starts a movement of such magnitude some one must stand at hand to take up his mantle and push the work with unflagging zeal. A great man cannot accomplish grand innovations without having great successors.

From the decay of ancient civilization to our own times the history of the insane has but repeated itself. In the middle ages common sense and science were dethroned by ignorance. Rationalism went to pieces and even the fragments fell down and vanished in the abyss of superstition. In such a benighted environment science could not thrive and all that had been done for the insane was completely lost. The insane fell into the clutches of superstition and mysticism and literally and figuratively sank into the hands of the devil, whence they were plucked forth by science centuries later through the Pinels, Tukes, Chiarugis, Daquins and ultimately placed in enlightened hospitals through State care agency and the labors of Esquirol, Foville, Guislain, Tuke, Conolly, Jacobi, Ferrus, Rush, Virgilio and Pisani.

The fate of the insane in the middle ages was simply hideous. They wandered about "possessed of Devils," without home or habitation, with everyone's hand against them and no choice between the Scylla of public cursings and the Charybdis of the care of their relatives. For we well know that *private* care of the insane, as it is liable to be in all times, is a species of private hell.

Things even came to a worse pass than this, the insane were not even accorded the saving grace of being considered human beings. They were not at times even taken to be men possessed by devils and fiends, but were held to be a different species, a set of animals or positive incarnations of devils taking on human guise. The atrocities which such a belief would entail upon the insane are hard to describe.

It is needless to dwell upon these things were it not to show that we cannot possibly expect progress in the care of the insane without fostering the scientific study of insanity.

Truly nothing was spared the insane from the brutality of the jailers armed with sticks and dogs, and the spittings and mockings of the multitude "for whom the sight of the misery of the insane became an object of amusement and recreation," up to the administration of noisome decoctions, rivaling the witches broth in Macbeth. One of these was Venice treacle, which started in with the flesh and broth of vipers, and then passing through sixty-two other ingredients, including all manner of disreputable weeds and filthy roots, strove for final absolution by tapering off with Canary wine and honey.

One redeeming feature of gentleness of humanity is the care of the insane of this age by the monks. While the monks could never free their minds from the belief that the insane were possessed by devils and fiends, compassion dwelt in their hearts, and their "*Exorciso te*" and "*Vade retro Satanus*," after New Testament teachings, were more kindly exorcisms of the devil than flails, stones, bludgeons and stakes. Churches and Holy wells accordingly often furnished a refuge for the insane.

Let us drop the curtain upon the times when the *quasi* religious man hardened his ignorance into contempt and vindictiveness at the sight of a Kepler explaining the pathways of the planets, of a Galileo elucidating the laws of mechanics, or of a Pinel smiting off the gyves of the insane. His enmity has long since smouldered into ashes, and out of them have arisen the beneficent hospitals of our own times; for meanwhile science had been slowly resurrecting

* Most undoubtedly the insane contributed the majority of victims to this evil torture. The vaporings and incredible feats which the paretic proclaims and the systematized delusions in certain other forms of insanity must have furnished abundant ease of conscience for the bigots of such times to torment lunatics as witches or devils. The doings of religious maniacs and melancholics must also have furnished sufficient blasphemy to merit torture and death. We can hardly believe, however, that it made much difference with the insane, whether they were called witches or "lunaticks."

from the tomb of the dark ages, and had chosen men of Philip Pinel's stamp as her apostles to deliver the insane out of bondage. No one with even a most languid interest in the terrible history of the insane or in their present welfare, can fail to be interested in the character and doings of Pinel.

The story of Pinel has often been told, but I trust that the moral I have in mind, in repeating a sketch the history of the insane, will not stand out any the less boldly by rendering the account again.

Pinel's work, unlike that of Hippocrates and Aurelianus, was enduring because he had the good fortune to have a successor like Esquirol. The secret of Pinel's power lay in the fact that he was an apostle of science. He had that which few, if any, about him possessed—an elementary but scientific knowledge of insanity. Beside this, he had the energy and courage to defend his beliefs against the pseudo-scientific and social prejudice of his time. He saw that the insane did not belong to a different species, but that they were human beings afflicted with a disease of the brain; that they had to be considered as patients, and receive medical care and treatment in hospitals like other human beings afflicted with maladies elsewhere in the body. Pinel's good fortune was his inspiration by science.

Toward the close of 1793, Pinel, who was physician at the Bicêtre (the great French prison for the insane), could stand the sight of things there no longer. He went to one of the leaders of the French Revolution for authority to take the irons off the insane. "His demand was bold, for he ran the risk of attracting the distrust and suspicion of men always disposed to find everywhere plots against themselves." In fact, the suspicion immediately betrayed itself in Couthon's reply:

"Citizen I shall go to-morrow to Bicêtre to inspect it; but woe to thee if thou hidest the enemies of the people among thy lunatics."

The man kept his promise, and arrived next morning at Bicêtre to examine the insane himself in detail. He soon tired of the monotony of the pandemonium of screams and yells, and the clanking of chains echoing from the damp and filthy cells, and, turning to Pinel, said, "Look here, citizen, are thou insane thyself, that thou wilt unchain such *animals?*" "Citizen," replied Pinel, "I am convinced that these lunatics are so unmanageable only because they are robbed of air and liberty, and I dare hope much from the opposite means of treatment." "Well, do with them what thou likest, but I am afraid thou will be the victim of thy presumption."

Pinel commenced work that same day. Had he not in advance taken all precautionary measures which such a step required, such as proper provision for the freed slaves, he would have failed. In less than a week he had freed more than fifty lunatics from their manacles. "Some were exceedingly dangerous, and among them patients who had been in chains for *ten*, *twenty* and even *thirty* years.*

Pinel stayed two years at the Bicêtre, encountering plenty of the pigheaded opposition of ignorance, but he had the satisfaction of seeing his efforts crowned with success. The excitement created by bad treatment gave way to quietness and improvement in the patients, and tractability replaced tumult and disorder. Everywhere he went, light, air and decent food came. Promenades and workshops arose to divert into wholesome trends the

* Dr. Pargeter in 1792 says that the festerings of these manacles and cords at times actually destroyed the flesh of the extremities. In one case where the jailer had tied the patient's legs with cords, when removed, these had so lacerated the integuments, tendons and ligaments, that gangrene took place.

disordered energy of the insane. Jailers were forced to discard their sticks and dogs and had to become attendants. In short, Pinel forecast the modern hospital for the insane.

Pinel then went to work at the Salpâtrière, another large prison for the insane at Paris. Again he met with blind, malignant opposition, but achieved success in the end.

Seldom, if ever, do strokes like Pinel's make their force felt as soon as it would be expected. *Vox populi* is often not *vox Dei*, but *vox ignorantiæ*. For the people are ignorant, and ignorance fights desperately against knowledge and science.

Without detracting from Pinel's glory it would be unfair to overlook the work in Germany, England and Italy. In Germany, in several places, Pinel's work had already been accomplished. As early as 1773, no lunatic was allowed admittance to the asylum at Berlin without a medical certificate. In 1785, at Frankfort-on-the-Main, a hospital of the enlightened type existed, and also at Lubeck (1788), and at Brunswick (1793). Berlin started one in 1784.

The reason for this advance in the care of the insane by Germany is not hard to find. The Germans foster scientific research; they have found out that it pays. Science is substantially encouraged by the government, and economy, strength, prestige and humanity are the returns. Amid such a splendid galaxy of names as Gall, Spurzheim, Haller, Burdach, Reil, Oken, Jacobi and Nasse it could not be otherwise. Observe, too, how, at the beginning of the century, Germany was taking means to sow broadcast a general knowledge of insanity, that it might not be immured or become narrowed within the asylum walls. We find that domiciles for the insane were built near the universities, where scientific investigation of the insane might be broadened out and an understanding of insanity brought to the general practitioner by teaching the medical student.

Dr. P. M. Wise, the president of our State Commission in Lunacy, has, in his recent address before the New York State Medical Society, struck the keynote of this same appeal to have a wider appreciation and teaching of insanity in our own country, especially when, in these days, we are stepping across the threshold of a new epoch in scientific investigation of insanity which bids fair to make a revolution in the progress of psychiatry.

Note, too, Germany's foremost attitude in arousing and keeping alive interest in mental science in her journals even at the beginning of this century. The magazine for Psychotherapeutics was started in 1805 and rehabilitated in 1808, with less pedagogy and metaphysic and more natural philosophy. A little later Nasse started a second journal which owed much to Jacobi, the Nestor of the German alienists who exercised a personal influence on the development of mental science in Germany.* In 1819 another journal devoted to the interests of the insane, appeared. In 1838 still another, and in 1844 Allegemenie Zeitschrift für Psychiatrie, which still continues.

Here are five journals devoted to the interests of insanity within the first half century. No other nation has a record like this. The influence of these journals on the progress of insanity has indeed been great.

* Homage is again to be rendered to Samuel Tuke, for his example influenced Jacobi who translated into German in 1822 Tuke's "Description of the (York) Retreat containing an account of its Origin and Progress, the Modes of Treatment and a Statement of Cases." (1813).

Germany's* example, then, is a fine monument for my plea of a state support of scientific investigation of the insane.

Italy was but little in the vanguard of Germany at the close of the last century. Chiarugi and Daquin had commenced reforming the asylum at Florence on Pinel's plans before the latter had begun his work.

In England, the work was taken up and continued by the Tukes at Bethlem and York retreat.

In the United States, the insane were at first subjected to the same abuses as elsewhere. But in spite of its early hardships and poverty, this country centering its efforts at Philadelphia managed not to be behind in the progress of humanitarian treatment of the insane.

As early as 1751, Dr. Thomas Bond put forth his efforts, seconded by Benjamin Franklin, for the establishment of an hospital for the relief of the sick poor and "for the reception and cure of lunatics." This hospital, too, recognized that insanity was a disease and that its victims were to be cared for and treated by physicians. It was in this hospital that Dr. Benjamin Rush gathered for twenty-nine years his experience that led him to suspect that much insanity arose from poisoning of the brain by the acute bodily diseases, an important point of view that has now come to the surface. It also should be remembered that the United States very early recognized the maxim of

* While Germany was in advance with a few institutions it is of course not to be understood that the length and breadth of the land was up to the same standard. This was the case in every other country struggling for the weal of the insane. One or two institutions were well in advance, but elsewhere they were sadly behind. In England, Tuke had enlightened Bethlem and York retreat, in Italy Chiarugi and Daquin did the same at the Florentine Asylum. In France, as we have seen, Pinel corrected Bicêtre and Salpêtrière. Throughout these countries the example was taken up very slowly. By her teachings, her journals, her hospitals, and the requirement of medical certificates, Germany had the lead.

Horace Mann that the dependent insane are wards of the State, a conception which led to their final redemption from abuse.

Twenty-four years passed by before Pinel's work advanced a single step. For Esquirol, his disciple, making an inquiry into the condition of the insane and their establishment in 1819, had occasion to write such bitter words as these:

"These unfortunate people are treated worse than criminals, and are reduced to a condition worse than that of animals. I have seen them naked, covered with rags and having only straw to protect themselves against the cold moisture and the hard stones they lie upon; deprived of air, of water to quench their thirst and of all the necessaries of life; given up to mere gaolers and left to their brutal surveillance. I have seen them in their narrow and filthy cells without light and air, fastened with chains in these dens in which one would not keep wild beasts. * * * This I have seen in France, and the insane are everywhere in Europe treated in the same way."

The second epoch in the progress of the insane is the period of passive indifference on the part of society. In several countries, in one or two institutions, the insane were released from the bondage of chains and on their way toward decent and humane treatment. But from the release of manacles to care and treatment in the hospital was a long stride, and unhappily a period of forty years from the beginning of the century awaited the insane in a second epoch of the indifference of society.* Very slowly indeed did Pinel's redemption make itself felt.

*In 1804 the law classed the insane with animals; thus the code Napoleon (Belgium, 1804) punished those who allowed "the insane and mad animals to run about free."

The insane were simply freed from their chains and nothing more. To any further progress society was indifferent. The insane were simply put out of the way, no longer actively tortured in the majority of instances, but merely gotten rid of. This was a period of sequestration, a negative mercy to the insane on the part of society, compared with previous times. After society had stowed the insane out of the way, where they could do no harm nor be heard from, this was the end of them. No one took the trouble to know whether justice and individual liberties were travestied, nor was there any pretense of medical supervision and treatment.

Accordingly the insane were stowed away in the iniquities of the almshouses, workhouses, and other rookeries, or confined with prisoners in jails. This was the epoch of social indifference, which occurred between Pinel's and Esquirol's times and the State care, culminating in the modern hospitals. This was the day of Bedlams, Pandemoniums and Madhouses, and over their doors might as well have been written the motto: "Who enters here leaves hope behind." This was not much of an improvement over the Infernos which Pinel found.

This kind of thing continued longer than we should expect. In Belgium, for instance, Guislain found it evil enough to suit the most pessimistic views of human nature. The physicians in the asylums held subordinate positions, under lay superintendents who were speculators, working the lucrative side of the thing. It must have been a fine thing to filch political money out of such poor devils as lunatics, and have their cost *per capita* reduced to seventy centimes a day. Most of the patients were under the care of their relatives, who were generally ready to believe anything of them, and treated them accordingly. Others fell into the clutches of mercenary Judases who bid against each other for the lowest prices. The patients were shut up in cellars, or small cells, with hardly enough to eat or drink, with chains and iron rings on their hands and feet, without the faintest pretense of medical authorization. Some, when brought out of these ratholes, arrived at the asylums in a dying condition. These iniquities were still going on in a civilized country in the years of the Christian era 1841 to 1850!

This condition of things should warn the custodians of the insane not to fall back into ancient practices of barbarism, by intrusting the insane, who are really diseased and have to be treated methodically and scientifically, like all other patients in hospitals, into the hands of the laity who are ignorant of medical science. Such a condition of things would tend toward a reversion to the old system of making the insane prisoners or slaves to people who would grind out of them whatever profit they could.

When the insane have recovered from their mental disorder, but not sufficiently to be able to stand the wear and tear on nervous energy in resuming the struggle for existence, it is most important to provide an intermediate stage of *after care* between their release from the hospital and their return to the activities of life. The plan of allowing the laity to have care of the insane except in the judicious *provision for after care* is opposed to the whole course of science which has taught us that *insanity is a disease and must be treated by physicians of special scientific training.*

The history of the succeeding epoch in the progress of the insane, is too familiar to need mention. Ferrus has much of the credit in initiating this most important step of State care of the insane in France during the latter portion of the first half of this century. Other countries independently took up the same work.

Within the last twenty or thirty years, with State care as the haven, and science as the beacon light, the insane have been guided into the refuge of enlightened care and treatment. They have been taken from the almshouse, the madhouse and pandemonium, from amongst criminals, and placed in enlightened hospitals. Dante's motto has faded from the doorway, and the hope of treatment and recovery is held out to them.

In our own State, we have good reason to be proud that our institutions are not in any way behind those of any other place in the world. The name of asylum redolent with so many hateful memories of the past has been erased and the word "hospital" symbolizing humanity and hope substituted.

The last word of the history of the insane in our own country cannot be written without paying tribute to the members of the first Commission in Lunacy of the State of New York, especially to its President, Dr. Carlos F. MacDonald, to the present Commission, as well as the superintendents of the State hospitals. The present progress in the treatment and welfare of the insane in our State is their achievement.

The history of the insane may be divided into four periods:

I. The Period of Revenge.
II. The Period of Indifference.
III. The Period of Humanitarian and Empirical Treatment.
IV. The Period of Scientific Study, Rational Treatment and Preventive Medicine.

The *first* period presents the spectacle of society under

the ban of ignorance, revenging itself upon the insane. This lasted some seventeen hundred years or more up to the times of Pinel.

The *second* shows the passive, indifferent attitude of society. This was the period of mere sequestration of the insane, witnessed in the first half of this century.

The *third* presents the more inspiring sight of the active interest of society in behalf of the welfare of the insane through legislation and the founding of hospitals for beneficent care and medical treatment. The third and present epoch we may designate as the period of empirical medical treatment. In this epoch the material welfare of the insane, such as their housing, comforts, amusements, moral and physical care, have reached a high degree of excellence.

The future and *fourth* epoch in the history of insanity will be the period of *rational* medical treatment and cure, and possibly by more radical measures in public medicine for the *prevention* of the increase of insanity. This will be based upon a more thorough understanding of the cause and course of the disease in any given case. This fourth epoch, the threshold of which we are crossing at the present time, is coincident with the **establishment of centres of scientific investigation**, in conjunction with systems of caring for the insane, in public and private hospitals. Science has hardly begun the broad and detailed investigation of the causes, origin and course of insanity. All this progress up to the present time has come about by the general march of science in medicine before even any detailed attempt was made to unravel the specific problems of insanity itself. How much more then, may we expect for the future when science will begin to use its present capacity and fitness to reach the very heart of the problem, the scientific story of the whole life history of insanity.

This new and fourth epoch in the history of the insane, launched forth by the stimulus of modern scientific investigation, will gradually point out the way and take into account the benefits of the *prevention of insanity*.

Unfortunately, the time is not yet at hand when these measures for the *prevention of insanity* can be at all extensively or successively applied. Public opinion is not yet reared up to the scientific truths as to the sources of insanity, nor of their menace to civilization and society.

In educational directions, a scientific basis for the phenomena of human nature should be taught earlier in the schools. The innate instability of the higher and self-controlling spheres of the brain and the proneness of these spheres to undergo retraction from other parts of the brain, under the influence of toxic and other pathogenic stimuli, and the concomitant phenomena of beginning insanity or degeneracy, should have an elementary and simple presentation in the school text-books on physiology. The same presentation should be made of the physical basis of heredity and the noxious effects of insufficient food supply and poisons upon the germ plasm and nerve cells. Above all, the action of alcohol upon the nerve cell should be impressed upon the minds of growing children as soon as they are able to assimilate such knowledge. The evil sources, such, for instance, as the dissemination of syphilis that lead to the worst and most intractible forms of nervous and mental diseases are here among us; we cannot overlook them; they are factors of life and the State must sooner or later face the problem of taking strong measures to counteract and mitigate them.

As already forecast by empirical experience, science,

even at this early stage in the new epoch of the scientific investigation of the insane, shows that in the case of an individual, without hereditary defects of the brain, the conditions for recovery are favorable. The probability that retraction of the arms of the nerve cell may dislocate them from their fellows, and cause corresponding dissociation of consciousness, synonymous with many phases of insanity, shows that no irreparable damage has occurred in the brain. Its mechanism is intact, but is merely, as it were, thrown out of gear. Each tiny cellular microcosm in the brain is intact, it has undergone no destruction, but a slender rift has occurred somewhere between the connection of the cells, and fields in the higher domains of consciousness are split off. There is no longer harmony, but discordance in the inter-relation of the spheres of higher consciousness.

The nerve cell itself may even undergo quite a train of organic changes without passing over into the bourne of destruction, hence the chances of recovery in a perfectly normal individual, undamaged by hereditary burdens upon his nervous system, are most hopeful. It remains for us to correct the process of retraction, which is a sign of deficient energy of the nerve cell, and the brain may be made whole again. Such a form of treatment worked out on strictly scientific grounds has actually been applied with successful results by one of our Associates at the Pathological Institute in a case of so-called double consciousness and has been based upon the principles of pure science, and premised step by step from a scientific investigation of the case lasting many months.

Science, however, cannot be expected to perform miracles in the cure of the insane. If insanity be taken in its early stages when the brain is free from hereditary defects, much may be accomplished and the view is hopeful. But if the beginnings of insanity have passed away, and are replaced by its later stages, whether in the individual or extended through a series of generations, the time has gone by when science might direct intervention. If a nerve cell is once destroyed, the damage is irreparable. A nerve cell is ordained with its functions but once during life, and is never replaced by a new one. If one, or two generations have damaged their nervous system and the germ plasm at the same time, and have entailed a heavily mortgaged cerebral estate upon their successors, the time for restituting the mechanism to provide for the lost energy of the nervous system has passed. Hence the constant plea of the scientist to those who have jurisdiction over the insane to seize the process in its beginnings, where it is less of a burden to the State, and more amenable to recovery, than in the final stages, hence the anxiety of the scientific student of insanity to look for the time when public opinion may at least put forth some few efforts in the direction of *preventive medicine* in insanity.

CHAPTER II.

THE PSYCHOPATHIC HOSPITAL.

The great importance, both practical and scientific, of apprehending the early stages of insanity, is obvious. The question is as to the means for this end. It is nothing short of a misfortune and an impediment to psychiatric progress in the large cities of this country and particularly in its metropolis, that no hospitals exist for the incipient and initial stages of insanity. The establishment of such a hospital is exceedingly important. It would encourage a better popular understanding of insanity and educate the rank and file of the populace to bring the insane earlier to the attention of the psychopathologist and psychiatrist. For the memories associated with the word asylum still linger in the popular mind. In spite of the enlightenment of the modern hospitals for the insane there is still an aversion in the lay mind toward bringing a patient to an institution for "the insane" until the case becomes serious, even dangerous. The asylum is thought of in the nature of a last resort and used under more or less compulsory circumstances. In these hospitals for initiary stages of mental diseases, placed in the midst of the great cities, many cases would be presented voluntarily and the custom of sending patients before becoming violent or mentally irresponsible would take root and grow. We should do all in our power to concentrate attention upon a wider apprehension of the beginning and acute cases of insanity. This can in the main be accomplished by educating and persuading the popular mind to the belief that in the treatment of the earliest phases of insanity lies the greatest hope of recovery, and that this hope dwindles more and more as the symptoms become more durable and persistent. The establishment of such a hospital would be a first and most valuable step toward the fulfillment of this educational influence of the importance of sending insanity in earlier stages than is presented to the ordinary hospitals for the insane. It follows likewise that the operation of such a hospital is an important factor in bearing on the *prevention of insanity*.

Dr. Peterson's name for this greatly needed institution —The Psychopathic Hospital—embodies its functions admirably. The name psychopathic hospital would sooner or later convey to the minds of the people a feeling different from that of the asylum. For in the commitment to the asylum, people believe that their relatives or friends are liable to be placed side by side, or at least in the same atmosphere, with the inveterate and doomed cases of insanity. This feeling certainly enlists sympathy. From this general repugnance to the asylum, and from the fact that the patients are put in a hospital for "the insane," thus branding them with the stigma of "insanity," naturally makes the family put off the evil hour of the diagnosis of insanity. The patient is retained at home, all hope is lost or the case becomes unmanageable. The psychopathic hospital in the metropolis would, in the course of time, largely do away with the prejudice that now holds back the early and favorable cases from proper treatment and study.

The meaning of insanity in the popular mind is most often crushing and conveys an element of hopelessness. If then these associations of the name are in a certain measure obstacles to psychiatric progress, we must take into account the popular feeling, especially as there are good scientific grounds for it and indulge it in a different and more hopeful conception of the early stages of mental disease. Let us substitute for the sweeping term "insanity" some equivalent, such as "psychopathy," which will convey to the lay understanding that the patients for this hospital are not yet insane in the popular sense, but are subject to a process, which if taken in hand, will prevent development into insanity. The sphere of the hospital is to seize the active percursor of insanity as well as the early stages of mental disease. The psychopathic hospital is for the reception of many patients which would not be ordinarily regarded as ready for commitment to the asylum. Yet from this very standpoint how valuable is its sphere in prevention and cure of insanity? *The psychopathic hospital is for the reception and wider identification of earlier, functional and more curable phases of mental diseases.* According to the idea based upon the principle of neuron energy as a law governing the progression of the phases of mental diseases* the insane fall into two great classes as regards hospital treatment and care. Broadly considered the first class would comprise those early phases of mental diseases corresponding to the *functional* mental maladies or *psychopathies*† should pass into the psychopathic hospital. The *second* class constituting the organic strata of mental disease or the neuropathies‡ and belong to the hospitals for the insane. This second class is composed of two groups. The first includes the cases whose symptoms correspond to degenerative and regenerative energy cycles of the neuron, while the second includes those cases manifesting symptoms of progressive degeneration and attended with destructive changes in the neuron. These two groups should be individualized in the hospitals for the insane.

The cases of the first class are amenable to recovery. Of the second class, the condition of the first group is less hopeful though recovery is not impossible; while the condition of the second group is hopeless.

The psychopathic hospital is practicable in the large cities. This distribution of insanity relative to treatment and care based upon the theory of neuron energy cannot be carried out in practice with fixed and absolute boundaries

* Vide "Neuron Energy and its Psychomotor Manifestations." ARCHIVES, Vol. 1, No. 1.

† The psychopathies exhibit phenomena concomitant with dissociation and aggregation of the neurons. Loc. cit.

‡ Loc. cit.

of the divisions. While the province of the psychopathic hospital includes the functional strata of mental and also certain nervous diseases, it should also provide for the cases entering the threshold* of the upper strata of neuropathic mental diseases. Certainly one great factor of practical importance independent of the advantages of such distribution for scientific study, is that the division brings the matter of expectancy of cure to the surface.

When one reflects upon the importance of studying and treating the earlier phases of insanity and its tendency toward preventive medicine in mental diseases, it seems really strange that the evolution of the psychopathic hospital in the large cities of this country has not been anticipated. The practical benefits of the psychopathic hospital are too obvious. The fact that the plan would bestow cure upon many patients who, left to themselves or their friends, would otherwise be committed to the asylum later in a much less curable, even in a hopeless condition, answers the argument of gain over cost and the practical utility of the hospital.

Abroad, particularly in Germany, almost every city and university town operates a plan of this kind in the institutions known as psychiatric clinics. In New York City it must be said to our disparagement that the only substitute—and perceiving the great purpose of such provision for psychopathies it is more a makeshift than substitute—is a pavilion at one of the public hospitals. Facilities for study at this place are few; here the cases are merely distributed to the various large asylums in the vicinity. As this pavilion is merely a centre of distribution it has neither theoretical nor practical therapeutic value. Whether or no such an institution should be

* Loc. cit.

undertaken wholly or partly by the State is a question out of my province, but the expansion of this pavilion into a psychopathic hospital is an imperative necessity.

From the practical issues let us turn to the value of such a hospital for scientific research in psychiatry. This may be summed up in saying that the very heart of the greatest problems in mental disease lies in the investigation of the cases entering the psychopathic hospital. The impetus to progress in psychiatric research from the scientific investigation of the cases in such a hospital cannot be overrated. Many who are providing the opportunity for the growth of scientific centres in connection with hospitals for the insane or whole systems of these hospitals are prone to think that the cases for investigation lie exclusively in the sphere of the asylum. This is a mistake. *Quantitatively the material for investigation in the asylum is indeed great, but qualitatively regarded the opportunities are few.* In the hospitals for the insane the majority of the cases are in too late a phase of the morbid mental process to be suitable for investigation. A single properly selected case in the psychopathic hospital where the morbid process and concomitant psychomotor phenomena are in an initial stage of development is worth more by far for investigation than hundreds of the average run of asylum cases. The investigation of such cases may furnish the key to great laws and principles governing the whole course of mental and nervous diseases.

The first thing in inaugurating scientific centres of psychiatric research is to find their sphere of investigation. This lies largely in the study of a class of cases which could be induced to enter the psychopathic hospital.

For the sake of illustration I venture to allude to the

scientific centre of the New York State lunacy system. This institution, while in intimate touch with the hospitals for the insane, is not incorporated with one of them for the express purpose of affording extensive scope of investigation. It is situated in the metropolis to seek material for the study in one of its most important departments—that of psychology and psychopathology. But without any systematic hospital provision for the psychopathies where to individualize and collect them, our opportunities for investigation in this most important province are limited and dictated by chance and accident. The study of these cases is not taken up by the university psychological laboratories for here investigation turns in the rut of routine scholasticism and is so immersed in the study of the psychomotor phenomena of the normal individual, the college student, that the great value of making progress in the knowledge of the normal phenomena by correlative research of the abnormal is unfortunately altogether neglected. The general practitioner sees many of these psychopathies. To him they are most often a sort of *noli me tangere* to be passed on to the specialist. From the psychiatrist they receive scant attention and ultimately fall into the hands of the neurologist who so little comprehends their nature and cause, but is ashamed to confess it.

Both the psychiatrist and neurologist have practically confessed inability to cope with these cases by merely identifying the phenomena in clinical groupings under purely descriptive names. As for the meaning of the psychopathic phenomena and the underlying morbid process they have caught but little more than a glimpse.

The ideal home of centres of psychiatric research is in the psychopathic hospital and clinic in the large cities where opportunities are also best afforded for the remainder of the diversified investigation of the institution. The psychopathic hospital would also exert a valuable influence upon the aim of such a centre of psychiatric research of bridging over the unfortunate gap in the scientific study between mental and nervous diseases.

The psychopathic hospital should include on the staff the general practitioner as well as the specialist, the psychopathologist, neurologist and psychiatrist; it should be the valuable meeting ground of both of these provinces or rather both departments of the same province. Under the influence of such a hospital an effort might also arise to seek out these cases instead of leaving the initiative of admission and committal of psychopathies and insanities to such an incompetent judge as the laity.

Stumbling blocks to the art and exiles from the science of medicine the psychopathies have been sadly neglected. Yet these same cases contain the greatest measure of knowledge for psychiatry, psychology, psychopathology, neurology and the science of medicine in general. The importance of collecting these cases in a psychopathic hospital and clinic for a wider, more accessible field of research is indeed great. Instruction in the combined psychopathic hospital, clinic and centre of psychiatric research would also be an important factor in medical education.

The beneficent influence of the psychopathic hospital is finely summed up in the closing lines of Dr. Peterson's address:* "A psychopathic hospital would accomplish a great practical good. It would be a boon to the many insane now gathered daily into a pavilion at one of our

* Inaugural address to the New York Neurological Society, May, 1898. Journal of Mental and Nervous Disease, June, 1898.

hospitals merely for distribution to various asylums. In such a hospital many cases could be treated and cured, thus avoiding transfer and commitment to asylums. Medical students and special students of psychiatry would profit from the convenience of access to the psychiatric clinics and the young graduate would enter upon practice with some definite knowledge of insanity and its treatment. But the greatest value of the proposed special hospital would undoubtedly be the opportunities afforded for those aggregate studies by many specialists which are destined one day to discover the origin and cure of many of the psychoses and incidentally to unravel some of the mysteries of mind."

Chapter III.

THE ASYLUM AND SCIENCE.

Turning now to the organization of research work in psychiatry, we must emphatically point out the fact that scientific work along the old routine lines of one-sided investigation of insanity, would be nothing but a snare and delusion; it would be a loss of time and labor; it would be an utter failure, barren of actual scientific results.

The one-sided scientific investigation of insanity by the microscope alone is not liable to yield results which a comprehensive study is naturally bound to bring about. It is equally safe to say that a restricted provision for scientific work on insanity, along the beaten track, followed for the last ten or twenty years, would, in a very short time, become effete.

The general impression seems to be not only among the laity but in the medical profession at large, and even in that branch of it which deals with the insane, that all that is necessary for scientific investigation in unravelling the life history of mental diseases, is to bring into the asylum microscopes, certain complicated machinery for cutting thin slices of brains, an assemblage of aniline dyes to stain these slices, and a goodly assortment of various sized bottles and jars for the preservation of the brains. This is a sadly mistaken notion of the way of investigating insanity. It has been done over and over again in the past twenty years at the hospitals for the insane, and the results toward advancing psychiatry were not only highly disappointing, but the plan has actually wrought harm.

Fettered by the incompetency of clinical methods of investigating the living patient, psychiatry turned for scientific light to the study of the dead through the microscope. Thus, while in the living patient were hidden great scientific truths and vast material for scientific discoveries which might have inaugurated new trains of thought and revolutionized whole departments of inquiry, the psychiatrist was unable to reap the benefits by reason of the inadequacy of his methods of investigation.

These methods are based on a wrong plan and an insufficient conception of the great comprehensiveness of the phenomena in insanity. The methods are of the clinical kind, adapted for observation at the bedside in ordinary general diseases of the body, but so utterly unfit for the study of mental symptoms that one can hardly expect to catch so much as a glimpse of the real nature of these phenomena. One may say that where inquiry by these kinds of methods leaves off a large part of true scientific research in psychiatry begins.

Thus psychiatric research is turned aside from one of its most important domains and nearly the whole burden of the work is cast upon the microscope. In this way, save to the few bolder minds, the inspiration of the whole scientific side of psychiatry is dwarfed and bound up in the work of the microscope and its accessories. It seems strange that so noble, so comprehensive a science as psychiatry should be circumscribed to a single unaided branch of scientific research as pathological anatomy by the methods of the microscope. But it is still stranger that this unaided branch of investigation should have been in itself circumscribed to the last degree. If the microscope is used broadly and with scientific reflection; if it is co-ordinated with many other branches of science, the research is most important in psychiatry. But in psychiatric investigation it seems as if mental vision instead of expanding as the lenses grew higher, diminished its scope of field hand in hand with that of the lens. Microscopical study in psychiatry has been made synonymous with specialized pathological anatomy of the nervous system. In fact, so specialized and restricted is this study, that what is gained in accuracy and minutiæ of facts is more than outweighed by a loss of comprehension and appreciation of their value.

This study is of a topographical nature. While it renders a conscientious account of the distribution of gross terminal changes in the brain in the last and destructive stages of mental disease, the detection of the early phases and of the processes underlying the whole life history of certain classes of insanity are entirely beyond its scope. Thus the pathological processes in the great mass of mental disease are ignored. Such a study again disregards co-ordination with pathological processes in the lower parts of the nervous system concomitant with nervous diseases. Pathological anatomy of nervous diseases presenting a simpler set of conditions for research should be intimately linked with and constitute the stepping stones to apprehension of patho-anatomical processes in mental diseases enveloped as they are by far more difficult conditions of study. Worst of all, however, is the fact that this investigation utterly neglects any philosophical correlation of morbid processes in the nervous system with those occurring elsewhere in the body. This seemingly constitutes the "speciality" of "specialized pathological anatomy of the nervous system"—to hold aloof from the light of analogy with the operation of the great fundamental laws which govern pathological processes in the whole body uniformly. This specialized study, not only in psychiatry, but also in neurology, has come to such a pass, that the nervous system seems to be regarded as something apart from the rest of the body, as if subject to peculiar pathological processes of its own.

This is indeed a puny effort to fathom the depths of so profound a science as psychiatry. Through this specialization its field of inquiry was isolated and the range of the intellectual sphere of the science correspondingly narrowed. This extreme specialization fastened itself upon psychiatry and blighted its genius. It rebuked that boldness of conception which diversity of study alone can bestow. Science has two sides; the mechanical side of merely gathering facts and the intellectual side of evaluating the facts and discovering the laws that underlie them. The discovery of laws, principles and generalizations is the true and highest function of science and constitutes the spirit of scientific progress; whereas if attention be wholly concentrated upon the mechanical side, science comes to a standstill. Many, however, confound the mechanical with the intellectual sphere of science. They are prone to think that the mere mechanical work of gathering facts is synonymous with the intellectual work of co-ordinating the values of the facts. This constitutes the great danger of specialization in science. This restricted plan of research fastened its view upon a single point and neglected the vast horizon of psychiatry. The little gain in new facts is really a great loss in the range of scientific thought.

In this way it has happened that psychiatry is behind all other branches of medicine both as to valuable facts and scientific theories; it even lacks speculations and hypotheses, the fertilizing germs of scientific progress. In this position many aspersions have been cast upon psychiatry. It has become a target for querulous demands for more rapid development than the organic laws of its growth would permit. It has almost become a fashion to attack psychiatry and complain that it has lagged behind all other medical studies. This criticism comes from the votarics of other departments of medicine, and among them prominently the neurologist, who immersed in his own peculiar limited and to him all important science forgets that the progress of psychiatric research is dependant upon advances in his own department. In fact the neurologist, "normal" psychologist and the "specialized" pathologist of the nervous system are the very ones to be blamed for the narrowness of the horizon in their own sciences and the supercilious air with which they regard the investigators of abnormal mental life. Well may the psychiatrist turn to these people and say: "And why beholdest thou the mote that is in thy brother's eye, but considerest not the beam that is in thine own eye?"

It seems to me that the sort of criticism coming from the neurologist, normal psychologist, specialized pathologist, etc., is shallow and even foolish. For what is the use of elaborating that which is perfectly obvious? Surely the obvious thing in the progress of psychiatry is that being the greatest, the most difficult and comprehensive of all medico-psychological sciences it must necessarily be the last to begin its progress. The psychiatrist has quite properly ignored this sort of criticism. At times, his just resentment has been aggravated, for he knows the greatness and difficulties of his science. Baffled in wresting out its truths without being discouraged, defeat quickening his resources, he has created the science and done all that could be done towards its advances. Yet in the midst of this he must needs suffer attacks from those who labor in a mere tributary science, stepping stones to psychiatry. He has had to hear criticism from the very ones who have held psychiatry in check by not developing or correlating their departments of research sufficiently to be of service in the difficult and comprehensive domain of psychiatric research. The psychiatrist has been in the position of Haüy, the great father of modern crystallography, whose means of observation were so rude that subsequent generations of crystallographers marvelled that he could have founded the science with such imperfect methods.

Perceiving the greatness of psychiatry in the past, realizing that the present is about to unfold its grandeur, and beholding psychiatry in the future as the queen of the neuro-pathological and psychological sciences, it is far from my thoughts to share in this conventional kind of criticism. If, therefore, in this text, I have protested against the inadequacy of the present plan of psychiatric research, it must be clear that this has been done in order that I might, according to my measure, substitute a larger, broader plan of the correlation of sciences in psychiatry which must surely encourage thought, scientific power of the imagination and engender progress. Even now the genius of psychiatry like the fabled *genie*, unloosed from the vial, is gathering into form, the haze is beginning to take on the stature of a giant among the medical sciences, and they who have carped at its growth, will be quick to render homage to its future grandeur.

While to many it may seem unnecessary to go into details respecting the inadequacy of isolated microscopic work in insanity—for the inefficiency of this present restricted method of microscopic research in psychiatry must be well recognized—nevertheless three reasons urge the discussion of the subject.

In the first place this restricted method is inadequate because it can only contribute to the mechanical side of science, it will do little more than heap up facts. *The restricted use of the microscope in psychiatry can only give microscopic results.*

In the second place, and here I think that others who are endeavoring to build up centres of psychiatric research will see the force of the argument, this restricted plan must be rooted up and its influence cast away before we can have the freedom and means to substitute the broader plan of the correlation of science in psychiatry.

In the third place, this restricted method benumbs the whole intellectual sphere of the science of psychiatry; it discourages originality and genius, the discovery of laws, principles, and deductive forecasting of effects.

Some years since in discussing the future progress of psychiatry and neurology, a distinguished psychiatrist and neurologist said to me: "We seem to have gone as far as we can. Every subject whether in neurology or psychiatry seems exhausted. There is nothing new to work at, or nothing to add to the old things. The microscope fails to give any new light." If this restriction of the investigation of both mental and nervous disease to the so-called clinical methods, and to the specialized pathological anatomy of the nervous system had produced such a gloomy impression upon a man of note, what must have been its effect upon the young observer entering either of these provinces in the fullness of enthusiasm for research. Certainly the effect would be to chill scientific imagination and flatten originality and genius. The stress of the restricted conception of work would drive him into the beaten track without his stopping to reflect upon broader plans of work. He would dig out a few more facts at the extremity of this narrow avenue of investigation and probably get the belief that this was accomplishing the true aim of science.

Since that time two great and powerful methods of microscopic investigation have come into use in neurology and psychiatry. From this it might be argued that the restricted plan of this specialized microscopic work in neurology and psychiatry was right; that it merely lacked improvement in methods. It is perfectly true that these two methods (Golgi's and Nissl's) afford a startlingly wider range of facts in the nervous system than we had hitherto dreamed of. But of what use are facts unless we appreciate their value? There must be something more than the microscope and the ability to work it. There must be *mind* to put a value on the facts. And for the mental evaluation of the fact there must be diversity of scope and the light of analogy that comes from a grasp of more than one limited department of research. If the microscope became so perfect that we could see molecules in the nerve cells, its unaided work would never give us the complete insight to the phenomena of thought, either normal or abnormal. I think the whole conception of the exclusive restriction of psychiatric or neurological research to the clinical methods and the specialized pathological anatomy of the nervous system by the microscope is wrong and inadequate.

For considerable time the thought has been growing on me as to the great importance of fields between several of the departments of neuropathological and psychiatric research. It seems to me that the investigation from these "*intermediate fields of science*" is what is most needed at present to counteract the drawbacks of specialization. Briefly stated, what is principally needed to grasp the great comprehensiveness of psychiatric research is the bridging over of psychiatry, psychology, neurology and pathological anatomy. If this union shall be accomplished in the newer science of psychopathology there will soon follow a *renaissance* in all of these branches of research. If then I have noted certain shortcomings of the asylum methods of psychiatric research, it is to measure the better the great benefit and inspiration to psychiatry that must surely follow the research conceived by a federation of sciences.

If a restricted mechanical plan of microscopic work were the right way to investigate the nature of insanity, it would be comparatively easy to write the stereotyped report of the microscopes, machinery and glassware bought, interspersed with prophecies as to what was going to be done with these things in clearing up the mystery of mental diseases. A list of autopsies by the hundred might have also been added presenting the conventional statistical arrangement as to age, race, sex, mania, melancholia, paresis and dementia, and the tabulation of the spots of softening, atrophy of convolutions, thickening of membranes, blood vessels, etc., or other gross signs of wreckage of the brain.

The mechanical method of applying the microscope would make things go smoothly in establishing laboratories for psychiatric research since it minimizes the burden of thought and scientific reflection.

The time has not arrived, nor will it ever come, when the scientist can be replaced by the mechanician and scientific thought by machinery.

Were this the way of investigating scientific problems of insanity, we would have simply had to carry the microscope into the asylum. There would have been no need of making such frequent explanations to the visitors of the Institute, in answers to their surprise of not finding such an institution centered in one of the hospitals for the insane, and confined to the *direct* study of the objects of its research, the brains of the insane.

The impression that scientific investigation of mental diseases is shooting wide of the mark and not attaining its object unless confined to the study of the insane themselves and their brains, seems deeply rooted in the minds of not only the laity, but also of the self-contented, routine-working, unreflective pathologists and psychiatrists. It makes at first, one blush, then uneasy, and finally simply bored when one has to reiterate to many a would-be scientific specialist, the same obvious elementary reply to the puerile question: "What has this to do with insanity?" when one man is observed at a desk, patiently studying the workings of the nervous system of the cockroach; and another is seen experimenting upon a perfectly sane individual and producing artificially some interesting departure from the normal operations of the mind, or a third investigator is inducing artificially a poison into the nervous system by an experiment on one of the lower animals; or a fourth investigator is watching the effects upon the nervous system of some ordinary disease of every-day occurrence, like typhoid fever, dropsy, or pneumonia. The time has not come, nor will it ever arrive, when any one can expect to understand normal or abnormal operations of the mind, by simply gazing through the microscope at the brains of the insane.

Fortunately this narrow conception of restricting the vast domains of psychiatric research to mechanical microscopic work has not been allowed to govern the planning of the scientific centre for the insane in the State of New York. The guardians of the State System of Lunacy have foreseen the advances that may be made by properly conducted scientific investigations of the insane, and have sanctioned the plan of departing from the beaten track.

There is but one way ever to expect success in the scientific study of the insane, and that is to conduct such investigations from a comprehensive and many-sided standpoint. This is perhaps more necessary for insanity than for any other subject that science deals with. What we want is an intelligent, methodical study of facts, phenomena, inductively collected observations and experiments, aided by the cautious but indispensable use of theory and hypothesis.

Scientific investigation of mental diseases must be unshackled from the narrow circumscribed conceptions which have so long governed it. Psychiatry must be freed from the confines of the asylum walls. The research must be broadened out and brought to bear on a great many problems which cannot be found within the asylum. The investigation must be brought forth into the outside world, and be applied to the great and varied number of phenomena which lead up to an understanding of the *sources* and *nature* of insanity.

The difficulty with the investigation of insanity in the asylum, is this: Insanity does not develop within the hospitals, because the patients are brought there after the symptoms have developed and often gone far on the highway of mental derangement. As a rule the patient is not brought to the asylum unless his mental malady has become so well established that he has become mentally irresponsible. Now on the face of the matter, it is hardly sensible to expect that we can get an insight into the deepest problem of science—the mechanism of mind, its variation, its operation, its growth and decay, its normal and abnormal manifestations—unless we have the opportunity of studying such operations in their very birth.

The direct and exclusive study of the manifestations of the insane in connection with some one single method as studying the microscopy of the brain in the asylum is the poorest way of attempting to attain any real scientific results. Such study is always prone to become narrow, and forget the enormous comprehensiveness of the great and diversified standpoint of the various factors in the source of mental diseases. The point may be illustrated by a single example. Suppose a man born of three or four generations of alcoholic ancestors, with a hereditary deficiency of the capacity for elaborating nervous energy. He attempts to go through the wear and tear of life, with a minus sign set down against the energy of his nervous system by the abuses and profligacies of his ancestors,* and tries to make good that deficient energy, by artificial means. He drinks alcohol or uses other stimulants to supply this lack of

*Vide "Neuron Energy and its Psychomotor Manifestations."

energy. (This is the meaning of the "craving for stimulants" in many men). He increases the mortgage on his nervous system, a mortgage started by his ancestors; and the penalty is ultimate bankruptcy of the capacity of the working power of his brain. He hovers on the borderland of insanity for a time, and is finally brought to the hospital. After spending months and years in the hospital for the insane, in a futile attempt to restitute a misspent energy of his nervous system, or eking out what unbalanced energy remains there yet, he finally dies, and often enough, by some intercurrent disease. It is perhaps unnecessary to go into details to show how futile it is to trace the life history of the patient's cerebral events with their parallel psychic manifestations, when we are given only the last paragraphs of the final chapter to work out the narrative. The task is simply impossible. One may as well go blindfolded through the first nineteen miles of a twenty-mile pathway, full of detours and devious turns, and then attempt to recount its topography and windings by going through the last mile without the blind. Yet just such work is being attempted all the time, and little good does it accomplish, in adding to the store of real knowledge of the why and wherefore of insanity.

It is perfectly true, in the case just cited, that with the microscope a number of changes may be found in the brain structure. As a matter of fact, they have been set down with much precision, according to the development of the methods of microscopic investigation at the time of record. The literature of insanity contains plenty of descriptions of alterations in the brain, in old inveterate cases of insanity, where mental disease has converted the edifice of the mind into a mass of ruins. When now the question comes up, as to what these changes mean, and the vital query as to the significance of these changes indicative of wreckage of the brain, then the same literature and the same observers remain silent. When it comes to the essence of the whole problem, the *meaning* of the changes that are seen under the microscope, the more important task of rising above the facts to their interpretation, of reflecting on the causes and course of these changes, remains almost wholly unaccomplished; in short the whole history of the psychopathological processes is sadly wanting, the very thing we wish to know. The conception and method of restricted microscopic work in psychiatry are fundamentally wrong. The most that such observations can point out is that the brain has gone to ruin, and this anyone with sound sense might well enough infer without taking time and trouble to pore into the microscope. The tremors and unsteadiness of the muscles, the unfaithful conveyance of messages from the outside world, into such a man's disordered brain, the insurgent gamut of his passions, the brutal and unbridled fury of his loosened sub-consciousness, and finally, the imbecile babblings indicative of the severance of the connections in the lowermost parts of the brain, all proclaim the ruin of the brain even to the most casual observer without using the high power lenses.

I dwelt upon this case, because in the minds of many this is the kind of material and the aspect of the problem that is to be given to the scientist to unravel some of the mysteries of insanity. In other words the selections are to be made in the asylum as to the mode and manner of carrying on scientific work. The discrimination and choice of the problems and the study by the microscope were hitherto directed by asylum men. This, at first glance, seems quite natural. The asylum physicians are to tell the scientist what to do, and how he shall work, how to use his materials and problems. This would seem a delightfully simple solution of the whole question—for by far the most arduous work in science is not in the material but in its mental sphere. The mental side of science is the master which governs the mechanical work in the external world. The ability to attain conceptions guiding science in gathering and co-ordinating causes and effects; the operations of inductive and deductive reasoning; the ability to suspect, forecast and predict the operation of causes; the judgment in selecting the fit problems from the unfit; the guidance of investigation and observation; the fashioning of theory and speculation in the scientific use of the imagination; all these constitute the highest and true aim of science and also its most arduous sphere of work.

Unfortunately such a plan as this—the general guidance or control of laboratory investigation of psychiatry by the asylum—still prevails as a general rule. Asylum physicians are to pick out cases here and there, preserve the brains, send them to the scientific centre and have the material "worked up for publication and contributions to science." Plans of this sort may be "practical" but for the "theoretical" purposes of science they are not liable to engender and encourage progress.

If the scientist is to be under the direction and control of the asylum physicians, and is compelled to shape his investigation of the problems befitting their conception, and is to be restricted to investigation of such autopsy material as they may see fit to choose, his energy is liable to be crippled. It is easy to ask for results or plan out work for another, especially when we are more or less unacquainted with the enormous details and complications of the physical methods for investigation, and leave in the background the mental methods of science that such work requires.

One of the positive obstacles in bringing a scientific institution for investigation of the insane in working order is to be trammeled by worthless cases and useless material. Another difficulty is to have the fact realized that nine cases out of ten, and that ninety brains out of a hundred chosen at the asylum and sent to the central institute contain insuperable difficulties for investigation, and their study most frequently contributes nothing to the advance of psychiatry. Furthermore, when such brains are sent to the scientist, the constantly changing intricacies of the problems of preservation are liable to be ignored, for these are to be learned by experience only, instead of following a stereotyped set of rules. The brains are generally spoiled by being improperly preserved; they are quite liable to have been treated by methods of preservation which render them unfit for the application of the latest and most modern methods of investigation. The time has passed when one or two routine methods were used indiscriminately for all cases of patho-anatomical investigation of the nervous system. Science is now in possession of a great number of methods in this branch of research and only years of experience can determine the adaptation of the particular method for the case.

A difficulty very liable to be encountered in establishing laboratories or institutions for scientific investigation of the insane lies in the fact that internes and other members of the staff are rather generally expected to be able to plunge into the intricacies of scientific research without any preliminary training. Naturally the results are disappointing. For it is not sufficient to have a given theme of research planned out by the scientist, the work must also be entrusted to a man of scientific training. If scientific research is to be extended among the staffs of the hospitals at least one or two men in the hospitals should be chosen with regard to their *previous scientific training* and not merely on the basis of their capacity to do the clinical or official routine asylum work. For such work, excellent as it may be in itself, does not enable a man to carry on scientific research.

It is unfortunate for the progress of scientific investigation of insanity that psychiatric research work seems to be held so simple a matter that any one with a little training may launch forth into the successful accomplishment of investigating the pathology and psychopathology of the nervous system. If men in the hospitals are to do scientific work they should have a good, solid *foundation laid for this work by preliminary education* in their undergraduate and medical (and post graduate medical) curriculums. *A biological and psychological training* in the undergraduate courses giving a broad scope of reasoning over the facts in pathological anatomy, psycho and cytopathology is not only highly valuable but indispensable. The science of medicine should be more generally coupled with biology and psychology.

Medicine is an art, and by far the greater majority of physicians are practitioners of this art, and we must free ourselves from the popular belief of confounding the physician, the practitioner with the scientific investigator. One may be a scientist without being a physician, and one may be a physician without being a scientist.

If medical superintendents of the hospitals for the

insane desire the members of their staffs to join the work of the scientific centre, they should choose among the men one or more who have had special training in some particular line of research as, for instance, in general pathological anatomy, combined with a knowledge of normal histology of the nervous system, or in some other branch of research, such as cellular biology, physiological chemistry, psychology, psychopathology, etc. Only after these conditions are fulfilled is the extension of scientific work to the hospital staffs feasible.

With some general as well as special scientific training among the members of the staff scientific work can be extended into the hospitals most profitably. To ask the director of the laboratory and his colleagues to supply this foundation, to cast aside their own problems and give up their valuable time, the result of years of training, in teaching what should have been learned during the college curriculum, is not only to retard the development and progress of the laboratory, but to bring its activities to a standstill.

Within the past decade two methods (those of Nissl and Golgi) have been developed in the microscopic investigation of the nervous system which have been hailed with delight by the psychiatrist, as these powerful methods open up exceedingly valuable avenues of investigation in the pathological anatomy of mental diseases. It is singular, however, that the impression should gain ground among many psychiatrists that all that is now necessary for the members of hospital staffs to take advantage of this lately arrived and long delayed opportunity for advances in the difficult domain of patho-anatomical research of mental disease is to master the mere *technical details* of these methods.

To master such a method as Nissl's is a comparatively insignificant task, but to interpret the results gained by the use of the method is quite another matter. This involves a wide knowledge of cellular biology, general pathological anatomy, and, above all, of the *general dynamics* and *organization* of the nervous system.

Furthermore, it is mere mechanical work to array facts concerning changes in an individual cell or group of nerve cells in some instance of a mental malady brought to view by Nissl's or any other method. To attain the real aim of science, however, we should reflect upon the meaning of these facts, and above all endeavor to connect them with the changes in *function* of the particular cell or set of cells involved and to ascertain what part the diseased cells play in the general *organization* and *functional interrelation of various parts* of the nervous system.

Facts are the building stones of science. Many devotees of science never rise above the mediocre position of carting the stones from the quarry and dumping them in conglomerate heaps; they use their methods in a routine fashion and gather blindly and without reflection facts which are often trivial and worthless. The true scientist is like the architect; he must first realize the *purpose* and *plan* of the building; he must know the *value* of the material and *select* it with great care. The true scientists not only gather valuable facts but also worry about their interpretation and the laws which govern them.

Familiarity with the mere mechanical side of technical methods does not enable one to appreciate facts, nor does it give him a knowledge of the appropriate application of the methods.

In brief, to expect hospital men to accomplish scientific research in mental pathology with little or nothing more at their command than familiarity with one or more methods of technical investigation by the microscope gained by a few days or weeks of study in the laboratory is as sensible as to expect a student to understand and intelligently use a foreign language by drilling into his mind a few rules of syntax. Without general and fundamental knowledge of the subjects to which scientific methods of investigation are applied, the mastery of these methods places the scientific novice in much the same position as the patients afflicted with mindblindness who see perfectly well with their eyes, but are unable to recognize the things seen.

The director of the scientific institution and his colleagues should not be called upon to overcome scientific mindblindness. This seriouly interferes with the primary object of the whole scientific work—namely, the investigation into the laws of insanity. To achieve such work, the scientific standard of hospital men must be raised. It would be advisable that examinations of candidates for positions of internes and juniors should provide for the entrance or choice of men with the requisite preliminary scientific training to make feasible the extension of scientific work into the hospitals.

If a scientist is to investigate the problems of insanity, he must be left absolutely free and untrammeled in the selection of such work which wide experience has taught him to expect good results. He must not however isolate himself, but should be in constant touch with his colleague, the hospital physician, advise and collaborate with him.

Our statement of the truth as to the relation of science to the asylum should not be taken as embodying the faintest echo toward anything derogatory to those who devote their whole lives in treating and ameliorating through clinical studies, the welfare of the most difficult and trying subject in all medicine, the unfortunate and dependent insane. We ought, however, to acknowledge candidly that few, if any, can learn to accomplish the intricate duties of the treatment and welfare of the insane, grasp the clinical science of psychiatry, master in addition the details of other fields of scientific investigation of insanity, and keep abreast with the advances in all of the stupendous side issues which such investigation must necessarily involve. It lies beyond any one man's capacity to master two or more provinces of science in these days of specialization. Life is too short.

There are a hundred different ways of investigating insanity. How is any one who is not familiar with these methods and working with them every day, to exercise the discrimination as to which shall be used to carry out a particular kind of inquiry? The work of microscopic examination of the human nervous system at the present day, a single branch of inquiry in the scientific investigation of the insane, is a herculean task. In fact no one man working months even in a single case, can accomplish it. Such work has to be divided up among several investigators whose training in his own particular specialty embraces no short period, in order to avoid the pitfalls of error, which constanly beset the pathway of investigation.

There is no royal road to science, nor is there any single way of examining the brain. Several methods, each with all of its intricacies and variations, in most cases have to be used simultaneously. When the brain is once taken out of the body and put in one preserving fluid or another, to make it fit for the preparation of thin, almost diaphanous tiny slices, which are stained with various dyes, for microscopic study, we may induce plenty of artificial changes in this procedure, changes that have no existence in the brain during life. All these things have to be taken into account and nothing but actual experience, learning from our failures and mistakes, can guard against the pitfalls of error.

Moreover, when an insane patient dies of some intercurrent disease, such as pneumonia, fever or some other secondary malady, having no primary relation to his insanity, the poison of the intercurrent disease leaves its traces upon the nerve cells, and greatly interferes with the determination of the pathological processes correlative with the symptoms of insanity. Such cases are at present of little, if any value, for scientific investigation. A set of lesions have been superimposed upon the pre-existing ones in the brain correlative with the symptoms of insanity, and it is hard to discriminate between the two sets of changes. All this is not liable to be taken into account by those who in their eagerness and enthusiasm for more scientific light upon the mysteries of insanity are naturally prone to select cases like these for investigation.

Even if the brain were properly preserved; cut into sections; perfectly stained in a dozen different ways, and weeks of study embodied in writing in the descriptive composition style: that the nucleus of the cell is "swollen," its body is "shrunken," "cloudy," "pigmented" or "unduly granular;" that its granules are "too fine" or "too coarse," or that its tail (neur-axon) is "thickened" or full of "holes." What of it? What good does all this do, if during the life of the patient there were no observations or experimentation upon the psychomotor manifestations beyond such ambiguous descriptions as "semi-delirious," "semi-stuporous" or "partially demented." This is like reading a book by studying minutely through a microscope the shape, size and color of the letters without the attempt to penetrate into their combined meaning. The mere heaping up of facts without understanding them as little constitutes the function of true science as the conscientious counting of stars deserves the name of astronomy. Piles of ungeneralized and unclassified facts in science are often so much rubbish. Pathological anatomy is in need of interpretations of its masses of facts by the aid of biology, cellular biology and psychopathology. In fact, observations by the microscope form a relatively small and secondary part of psychiatric research. Its great sphere is the psychomotor manifestations themselves which little more than shadows across the microscopic field.

Cases at the hospital for the insane must be *critically selected* for study and experiment; their psychomotor manifestations closely studied by observation and experimental methods borrowed from the domain of psychology and psychopathology. Furthermore a progressive series must be found in which the definite phases of the psychomotor manifestations correspond to certain stages in the whole course of pathological process.

It is clear, then, that there are many drawbacks to the direct study of insanity in the loose and restricted way in which it is carried on at present. It is the *largest problem in science*, and it cannot be imprisoned within the asylum if we ever expect to find its solution; and the present time bids fair to justify such an expectation, provided the study of the problem be properly and broadly undertaken.

I am aware that it may sound sententious to speak in this way of the futility of the restricted method of attempting to study insanity directly within the asylum walls, but I cannot help pointing it out since it is the wrong way of solving the problem. Ninety-nine brains out of a hundred, the symptoms of which we are asked to explain by the microscope, are at present absolutely worthless for study. It is a mere waste of time.

Why is psychiatry in the rut in which we find it to day? Because, frankly speaking, as intimated in the subsequent text devoted to psychology and psychopathology in the next section, psychiatry has no appropriate scientific methods to work with in studying its field of inquiry—the abnormal phenomena of consciousness. The only methods which psychiatry has are *clinical* methods. These are appropriate only for investigating the phenomena of the *lower parts of the nervous system* and *symptoms of the body* and are wholly incompetent to investigate the abnormal manifestations of the *higher parts* of the nervous system correlative with abnormal states of *mental* life. The investigation of the bodily symptoms in insanity are of the highest value, because through the body we may attempt to correct disorders in the nutritive supply of the brain and restitute pathological expenditures of energy of the nerve cell, but in attempting to investigate *mental symptoms* psychiatry must use the methods of pathological psychology or psychopathology.

CHAPTER IV.

PSYCHIATRIC INVESTIGATION.

In the last chapter we have pointed out a very natural reason for the backwardness of psychiatry after other branches of medicine have made considerable and even brilliant advances. Psychiatry has had to wait until several tributary sciences, especially the science of consciousness—psychology—attained a considerable degree of development. At present these tributary branches have reached a growth and capacity to enter the service of psychiatry and its future is indeed grand. The story of the progress of psychiatry is simply the story of the progress of any other science. Every science, no matter how far it may be advanced, has had its infancy. So it is with psychiatry, and it would be exceedingly presumptuous to take the science to task, so to speak, because it is in an early period of growth. We must remember that this is one of the youngest departments of all medical sciences. It is only twenty or thirty, or at the outside, fifty years since psychiatry was recognized. The understanding of insanity was exceedingly late in emerging from the ignorance, prejudices and scholasticism of the middle ages.

It must be borne in mind too that the empirical development of the art of psychiatry was inevitable to herald the birth of the science. The material welfare of the insane, their recognition as wards of the State, the building of hospitals, medical care and treatment, had to be worked out empirically in their natural course, and all these experiences had to be gained as a starting point for scientific progress in insanity. The function of art is utility, that of science, ascertaining truth; the one seeks to control phenomena, the other gains foreknowledge of them. As knowledge and civilization advance, one of their greatest achievements is to replace the empirical faculty of control represented in the sphere of art by a scientific basis. In any branch of knowledge capable of practical application, art develops first and grows up to the limits of empiricism. Then science appears, replaces the empirical basis of art and continually expands and strengthens its power of control and utility by placing the predictive power of science at the service of art. Looking forward into the future, it seems to me that this is happening to psychiatry. The art of psychiatry has attained the limits of its (more or less) empirical development; the true science of psychiatry is now beginning to appear, and from now on will bestow on the art the fertility of a scientific basis.

Psychiatry has reached the limits of the methods used for the last twenty and thirty years. It has done all that it could in that direction. Future fields of investigation are perfectly barren, unless this science gathers new facts. This it cannot do unless removed from its rut makes use of methods which at present it does not possess, and is correlated with other affiliated paths of investigation in medicine, biology and psychology.

There is a right way and a wrong way of attempting to investigate insanity. The wrong way is to restrict the whole study of insanity to the brains of insane patients, long after all clues have disappeared from scrutiny. The wrong way again is to study the brain as though it were apart from the rest of the body and subject to peculiar laws of its own in the origin and course of disease processes. Investigators in psychiatry are liable to take but little heed of the advances and investigations in morbid processes which take place in other parts of the body, such as the kidney, the lung, or even the humblest constitutents of the organism, such as the simple tissues. The process underlying disease and its several phases which we call degeneration, inflammation, hyperplasia, etc., and wrongfully intimate as distinct entities, are of the same fundamental nature in these simpler organs and tissues as in the complex nervous system. Presented under simpler conditions for investigation in the simpler tissues and organs, the light of analogy is most important for the valuation of the homologous pathological processes underlying mental and nervous diseases. But many have fallen into the great danger of specialization in studying the pathological processes of the nervous system. For specialization coerces the attention to a single part and is prone to breed neglect of the relation of the part to other parts and to the whole. No one can expect to understand pathological processes in the nervous system by studying them in that system alone. To understand morbid processes in the nerve cell one must study them side by side with a knowledge of the cell in general, and correlate the study of the pathological anatomy of the nervous system with the general pathological and physiological laws valid for the organism as a whole. What is needed *is less* "SPECIALIZED" *and more* "GENERALIZED" *study of the pathology of the nervous system.*

If I were asked to give any one prominent reason why we have so little scientific knowledge of the life-history of insanity, I would say it is because of insufficiency of methods of investigation and its restriction, for instance, to the mere mechanical microscopical work on the brains of the insane. The enormous advances and revolutionary methods in the anatomy and physiology of the nervous system, in psychology and psychopathology, in cellular biology, and in the study of pathological processes in the body at large seem to have remained outside the pale of the asylum walls.

The psychiatrist seems to think in studying the scientific aspect of insanity, in investigating the patho-anatomical changes in the brain that he is dealing with something apart from the rest of the body, apart from every science except psychiatry and need not be concerned with general knowledge and methods which mark the enormous advances of the present day in normal and abnormal psychology or psychopathology, cellular biology, physiological chemistry, comparative neurology, general pathological anatomy, cytopathology, etc.

It might seem as though it had been intimated here that microscopic investigation of the brains of the insane in the asylums was of no use. This is not the point. The protest is against *exclusively restricting* the investigation of insanity to such a province. The investigation of the brains of the insane in certain critically selected cases at the asylum, under the guidance from beginning to end of a life study, of the methods of this field of investigation and of a correlated study with disease processes occurring throughout the body in general is of the utmost value. The only protest has been against this constituting the whole and exclusive field of scientific investigation of the insane.

No such restricted investigation can hope to do much more than to set down a few desultory facts in the ultimate chapters of the life-history of insanity, and even then with no explanation as to what these facts mean or how they have come about. As it is now, we are quite familiar with the gross alterations that go hand in hand with wreckage of the brain in old inveterate and terminal cases of insanity, but we know comparatively little of what these changes mean, and still less as to their relation to the production of the patient's symptoms during life.

While the undue subordination of the many-sided domain of psychiatric research to microscopical work on the brain is unphilosophical and restricted, this work in itself is extremely complicated and the value of a commanding view of its intricacies has not had as general an appreciation at the asylum as might be desired. In this branch of work there are dozens of radically different plans of investigation, and each one of these with its several technical methods and their variations and complicated details, has a specific and definite object to attain that no other method can give. It takes years of large experience with these methods of investigation to determine which one will subserve the best use; for one must plan ahead, from the very moment the brain is removed from the body, and apprehend, in a general way, the character of the disease process which is at work to choose the particular method of exposing its traces upon the nervous system. Very frequently provisions have to be made for the simultaneous use of several methods of investigation of the nervous system of any one particular individual taken at the stage of the disease which bids fair to yield interpretable results. Hence the great embarrassment which the scientist is constantly encountering in material sent to him for investigation is the fact that it is either placed in some fluid which is utterly unfit for the particular line of investigation or it presents some inappropriate phase of the pathological process.

In an institute for the scientific investigation of insanity, it is a bad plan to burden the scientist with autopsy material selected and preserved by any one who lacks the experience and training in the methods of microscopic study which alone gives discrimination as to which one of a great many methods is fit to use, and it is wrong to put the scientist to the impossible task of elucidating anything from such material. Yet, as a general rule, the rather elementary idea seems to have taken root that the operations of such a department are to be carried on by placing the scientists in its charge in the untenable position of investigating brains that are either unfit from the selection of the stage of the disease or impossible of investigation by reason of unsuitable preservation. It is unreasonable to suppose that any one can gain knowledge of the material best adapted for profitable pathological study or the intricate technical methods of this investigation without making it a subject of detailed and specialized study.

With the exception of interpreting the results of study of abnormal changes in the brain with the microscope, the preservation of the brain and other organs of the body is the most important datum in the whole investigation. For if the first steps in the investigation, the details of preservation for microscopic study, be wrong or inefficient, the accomplishment of the subsequent steps of the research is out of the question. The scientist must have complete control of the scientific work, and yet work hand in hand with his scientific colleague, the clinician.

The sections cut from the brain for microscopic study are but one-ten-thousandth of an inch thick, but the surface covers over one hundred square inches. It would, therefore, require the study of millions of these sections, which are generally but one-half the diameter of a penny, to make the microscopic examination of the brain in any given cases of insanity at all complete. The human nervous system has such a large volume and is so extensively distributed over the whole body that much judgment must be exercised in choosing the particular regions upon which to concentrate the bulk of the microscopical study. It lies beyond the capacity of a single observer to make a complete examination of the brain. It requires a force of several men to divide up the work within limits that can be accomplished. No wonder, then, that the work at the Institute, even in this single department of microscopic study of the brain, has to be subdivided and the results correlated weeks or even months after the investigation is started. In fact, in addition to the herculean task of examining the abnormal brain one must constantly have at hand sections from the same regions in the normal brain to measure and compare the changes in the abnormal brain.

Few realize that it takes years for an investigator of even the largest opportunities to collect material from the bodies of patients suffering with any particular form of disease, to correspond to all the phases in the pathological process of that disease. People seldom die in the great majority of diseases, until the process underlying the disease is well established, far advanced or has reached terminal, often destructive stages, so that we have no clue for tracing out the origin and course of the morbid process.

In a particular disease, for instance, we had to wait a number of years before any clue could be obtained to the origin of certain peculiar destructive canals running up and down the spinal cord. Several years after finding the terminal result, the beginning of the disease was seen, in which state patients exceedingly seldom die. But the beginning and initial stage of the disease was so different from the terminal and destructive alterations that the relation between the two was not recognized. Finally, within the past year, a patient happened to die in the middle stages of the disease, and now piecing all the stages together, we are able to record the pathological process underlying a hitherto unrecognized disease of the spinal cord. So it is with disease processes in insanity. If the brain is examined at some particular stage in the course of the disease, this does not by any manner of means tell us the whole story of the morbid process, it is a mere episode in the life history of the disease, a portion of a single chapter, which perhaps forecasts the next, but tells us very little about the preceding chapters. We have to trace the history of the early phases as we have opportunities of finding them, beginning at the first, but certainly not at the last, and working backward, a decidedly wrong order in such an enormously complicated problem as relates to the pathology of mental and nervous diseases.

The well nigh insurmountable obstacle of the direct study of insanity within the asylum is that the most difficult aspects of the problem are encountered. In most of these asylum cases the gap between the effect and cause is too great for induction to span the bridge. Nor, as a rule, can we put the materials from the asylum under our immediate control and experiment for varying the conditions indispensable to the inductive method. In studying the earliest phases of insanity these difficulties are greatly reduced. These earlier phases are nearer to the causal end of the morbid process manifesting itself in a series of successive phenomena amenable to control and experiment. By a series of experiments in which by successively varying the surrounding circumstances and then carefully noting the facts, undesired perturbations may be eliminated and principles and laws may be discovered. This accomplished we may use the laws deductively and descend to the facts, bringing more and more of them into harmony and within the fold of the law. After this stage in the investigation—the discovery of a guiding principle—the later phases of insanity, constituting the majority of cases in the asylum, may be more clearly understood. Finally, science being in possession of the secrets of the early stages and the predisposing factors of insanity will exercise its highest power of forecasting and controlling phenomena. This being at the disposal of psychiatry as an art, may yield practical therapeutic and prophylactic methods far exceeding our most sanguine expectations.

It is in the study of the early phases and predisposing and proximate causal factors of insanity that one begins to realize the comprehensiveness of the science of psychiatry and the enormous extent of its ramifications. It is here that the play of the correlation of many sciences comes into action.

We must proceed from the simple to the complex. The simpler aspects of the problems in insanity—simple only in constituting the scientific order of progression in the advance of psychiatry, but otherwise exceedingly difficult and comprehensive—can only be solved on the basis of a general comprehensive work. The work required for the investigation of these early phases include, for instance, the study of the architecture, cytology and functions of the normal nervous system; of pathological processes of the body in general and of the nervous system in particular under the influence of hurtful stimuli such as poisons, abnormal fatigue, diminution of food supply to the nerve cells; of the development of the brain both phylogenetically and ontogenetically. This study from the standpoint of phylogency and ontogeny is most important. For it gives an insight into the laws which govern the dissolution of the nervous system, the reverse process of evolution. *All mental and nervous diseases are manifestations either of the retrogressive process or of incomplete and defective evolution.*

We can realize now how meaningless and futile mere mechanical and microscopical work in psychiatry may become without correlative knowledge of the evolution of the nervous system and of the functional inter-relation of its parts. Without such study microscopic work in the nervous system is blind and does not know what to do; it gropes in the dark and labors aimlessly in the hope of making some valuable discovery by sheer accident.

Generally speaking, the organization of the nervous system in relation to function may be described somewhat as follows: The most supremely organized parts of the nervous system, the last attainment in man's evolution, the most precious part of the brain, which it has taken eons of time to evolve, which gives man his discrimination, his powers of ratiocination, his self-control, are the most unstable parts of the make-up of the nervous system. These higher and last evolved parts of the brain are prone, in the presence of pathogenic stimuli, to become dissociated from the remainder of the nervous system first and with their dissociation appear the first beginnings of unsoundness of mind. It may be seen, then, how absolutely essential it is to have the complete story of the evolution of man's brain, both in the individual and in the species, and to find out how this nervous system has been progressively built up, one part added after another, corresponding with higher and higher functions.

We may watch this in the development of species or in the child's brain. When the child comes into the world it has absolutely nothing to its credit in the functions of the nervous system, except the operation of that lower part of the nervous system which presides over the most fundamental functions absolutely necessary for the maintenance of organic life, such as respiration, circulation and a few reflexes. Little by little, higher and higher portions of the nervous system develop. Slowly and progressively the sense organs transmit desultory and uncorrelated messages of the physical aspect of things in the outside world. Still later the messages from the outside physical world are correlated in a simple and elementary form and a low grade of consciousness and recognition of things in the external world begins to dawn upon the child. Ultimately, by the use of the very highest parts of the brain which man possesses, the child learns to discriminate among these impressions and their correlations to the outside world, as to what is significant and as to what is insignificant. Still further along, as the child becomes older, by constant use and education of the supreme and highest part of the nervous system, he learns self-control and inhibition over the lower parts of the nervous system and higher and more complex forms of syntheses of consciousness.

These supreme centres of the nervous system, which exercise control and inhibition and a bridling of the lower parts of man's nervous system, which latter we share in common with the animal, are the last to ripen and mature in the education of our brains. The maintenance of this part of the nervous system requires constant vigilance and exercise all through life, and a great majority of people never completely learn to make these centres less unstable than they are bound to be through the laws of evolution. A whole lifetime does not suffice for great multitudes of people to gain sufficient stability of these centres by constant exercise and training. The consequence is that by over-fatigue, deficient nourishment, or by poisoning of the nervous system, a progressive dissociation and finally disaggregation of the nervous system occurs in the reverse order of its evolution. The highest and most complexly organized, and naturally the most unstable portions become dissociated first, as witnessed in *neurasthenia*. Then in a steady progression the dissolution descends to lower and lower parts of the nervous systems until in dementia and idiocy but little else than the most elementary systems of the brain presiding over vegetative and automatic functions are left-intact. This is in brief the epitome of the life-history of insanity.

As a contrast between the old and the new conceptions of investigating the scientific problems of insanity let us recur to the example mentioned in a previous chapter, where it is pointed out how futile and impossible it is to reconstruct from a few observations of the last few stages the whole life-history of the patient. Under the new conceptions of study, at our own Institute, for instance, the problem is being attacked from several standpoints. In the first place, we study the initial effects of alcohol upon the nervous system, which is not accessible to investigations confined to the asylum. We study first the exaggerated effects of alcohol where it has acted as a deadly poison, for instance in the brain of a case of fatal delirium tremens. The selection of such a case is not by any maner of means a simple matter. We have to select an individual dying of this disease in which we feel perfectly sure that the alcohol poison is not complicated with other diseases. We must find an individual whose nervous system has not begun to grow old. He must be an individual perfectly normal in all respects, so that we may be perfectly sure that what changes we find in the nervous system are due to the action of the alcohol and nothing else.

To obviate these difficulties, however, the problem becomes much simpler in the investigation of the direct action of alcohol on the nerve cells, by experimenting on animals. This is a much more satisfactory investigation in many respects than the study of the effect of alcohol on the human nervous system. For, in the animal, we can perfectly regulate the amount given, we can stop the experiment at any stage, either at the beginning, middle or the end, and study the brain cells at all stages during the action of the alcohol.

In the light of these studies the effects of chronic alcoholism in the human being may be studied with greater profit. Here we get an inkling of the premature senility which chronic alcoholism brings about in the brain. We witness the effect of a failure on the part of the myriads of tiny constituents of the nervous system—the nerve cells—in their capacity to store energy, which they receive in the food supply from the blood vessels.

Besides this, we investigate the phenomena of intoxication in an individual to whom the alcohol is given as an experiment. We give him memory tests, discrimination tests, study the quality and intensity of sensations, the emotional character of ideas, the disorders of associations, of judgment, and, in short, devise means to measure and recount the interference with the working power of the highest powers of his nervous system. Such experiments are highly important because in the phenomena of alcoholic intoxication we have a general outline reflecting all the phases of insanity. The highest and most precious portions of our brain being the last to become evolved and educated, are also the most unstable, and are the most ready to undergo dissociation under the action of noxious stimulants. Alcohol, accordingly, begins its dissolution of the nervous system at these very highest centres of discrimination and self-control. The dissolution of the nervous system progressively descends down to lowest centres which preside over respiration and circulation, so that finally in profound intoxication the whole nervous system with the exception of the vital centres indispensable to the life-being of the organism is in a deep sleeping state. If the poison by alcohol proceeds too far, even the vital centres are suspended and death ensues. Thus it will be seen that in this third line of study of alcoholic insanity, the whole broad domain of the evolution and reverse dissolution of the nervous system is involved, a field conjointly demanding the attention of both the psychopathologist and cerebral anatomist.

The same problem, from the standpoint of chemistry, is approached more closely in the brains of the habitual drunkard. We endeavor to bring the methods of chemistry to bear on this problem, to see what chemical changes occur in the nerve cell in its degeneration from the habitual use of alcohol. Hand in hand with all of these investigations, are studies of the normal nervous system by the microscope, which must go on for many years before we are perfectly sure of a standard of comparison to judge of abnormal changes in the brain. At the same time other investigators are at work peering into the workings of the nerve cell in some of the humblest living creatures. For the nervous systems of the lower animals are far simpler to understand. It is much more essential to arrive at some of the fundamental laws governing the workings of the nerve cell in some of the lowest creatures than to attempt to ascertain these truths in the most complicated form of the nervous system that can be found, namely, that of man.

I can only touch in the most desultory fashion upon the great number of pathways that have to be pursued, and the great many side issues of the most profound scope, which have to be taken into consideration, in studying the initial stages of insanity. But this is the only way we can proceed to study the more complex and advanced stages in the hospitals for the insane. This elementary sketch ought, at least, to show how many-sided the problem of insanity becomes when taken out in the outside world beyond the scope of hospitals for the insane. Such an illustration ought to show how enormously scientific investigation of the insane broadens out, even when we start at what is comparatively the simple end of the problem, namely, the study of the first phases of insanity.

To sum up the practical difficulties liable to be met with in establishing centres of scientific investigation of insanity they may be presented as follows:

1. The scientific centre must first identify and formulate its purpose and sphere of investigation; it must deliberately choose its plan before the building materials can be wisely selected; after this the laboratory or scientific centre must be given time to become equipped and organized and collect material for work; and also to apportion its general themes and special work among the members of its staff.

2. This work, from beginning to end, must take precedence of everything else and should not be interrupted by premature demands for the results of scientific work and for publications to be completed simultaneously with the organization of the laboratory, or by demands at any time for scientific research to be made to order or completed hastily.

3. The energies of the members of the staff must not be wasted in instruction that is unprofitable, or in imparting knowledge where a ground work of scientific training in general pathology, psychopathology and neurology is lacking. Instruction should only be asked when it can be

made profitable, in cases where a proper foundation has been laid previously. It requires years of instruction to supply this deficiency that ought to be made one of the requirements of entering the hospital if men are expected to do good scientific work.

If matters (2) and (3) be not held in the background pending the organization of the laboratory, or if all three of the subjects be attempted simultaneously it is quite certain that none of them can be done well, not to speak of the danger of seriously retarding the growth of the laboratory or bringing its energies to a positive standstill.

Fortunately all these drawbacks have not been encountered in the inauguration of the Pathological Institute of the New York State Hospitals. It has departed from precedent, and has been given the most cordial encouragement from its colleagues in the commission and at the hospitals, in insisting upon a broadening of the study of insanity from the modern standpoint of the correlation of many branches of science. Only through such encouragement have we been able to depart from the beaten track, and insist that the study of material within the asylums is not the whole essence of approaching the problem, and in fact constitutes but a relatively small part of the work. The scientific staff at this institute has not been hampered in the planning and direction of the scientific research work. Proper fields of inquiry are submitted to their judgment and trained discrimination. We have learned the value of the indirect study of insanity, of approaching it through a number of avenues, which, while not directly investigating the insane themselves, is infinitely more valuable at the present time.

The Institute has the opportunity of studying the conditions which lead up to the begininngs of insanity and of observing people before they arrive at the asylum. It has been permitted to study the effects of general bodily disease upon the nervous system, and has been situated in the metropolitan centre of the State, where it might be in touch with the acute general hospitals in the investigation of the nervous system in the great mass of ordinary diseases of everyday occurrence. Its energies are not wasted by being compelled to study material which some one has selected, who does not know how it should be studied or whether such study would yield results of scientific value.

The direction of the institute has been encouraged in planning for the study of the *evolution* and the *dissolution of the nervous system.*

Provisions have been made for the psychopathological investigation of the various dissociations and syntheses of consciousness in the abnormal individual as well as experimental induction of these phenomena of consciousness in normal men and even in animals.

The plan has been followed out in collecting material, the investigation which seems, at first glance, but slightly related to the elucidation of the life-history of insanity, such as the brains of the lower and lowest creatures; autopsy material from *nervous diseases*, in contra-distinction to mental diseases; and also developing stages of animal life.

The paramount value of facilities for *animal experimentation* for the conjoint investigations of the physiological chemist and the psychopathologist of the action of *poisons* upon the nervous system has been recognized.

A very essential factor in the general plan of the work of the Institute is the necessity of providing for and stimulating research work in the study of the effects of somatic or general bodily disease upon the nervous system. To subserve this purpose the Institute has been brought in touch through several of its associates with several of the large general hospitals in New York city, and thus has the opportunity of studying autopsy material and investigations from a psychopathological standpoint, particularly the changes in the nervous system associated with the great mass of general body diseases.

Thus we have provided facilities for investigation of the damage wrought upon the nervous system by the great host of general body diseases. This method of study, it will be seen, cannot be undertaken in the hospital for the insane. It must be followed out in the material from ordinary general hospitals and is most feasible in the large cities. The effects of the great mass of body diseases upon the nervous system are hardly at all known as yet, and most important are the results of future study in this field for the understanding of the changes in the brain going hand and hand with insanity.

The phenomena of insanity are manifold and their comprehension can only be grasped when viewed from many different standpoints—from the standpoints of many sciences. A co-operation of many sciences will bring forth a rich return of both theoretical and practical results. A many-sided, comprehensive, scientific investigation of insanity is at present an imperative necessity. We are on the threshold of a new era in the study of the nervous system in both its normal and abnormal manifestations. The inauguration of this era not only requires specialization but also interaction of the lines of research. Different branches of science must be co-ordinated and focussed together as a search-light on the mysteries of mental diseases. They must all work hand in hand.

They must be linked together and correlated, otherwise the whole aim of the work is defeated; the investigation will become one-sided and restricted, and what few facts are gained will not be open to comprehensive interpretation.

In accordance with the tenor of these prefatory remarks several departments of research ought to be established at a scientific centre for the investigation of insanity. If I may take the liberty of alluding to the scientific centre of the New York State lunacy system—the Pathological Institute of the New York State Hospitals—we may now review the purpose of these several branches of science as planned in this institution and observe the general aim of the special and combined work. Such a review, however, must be made exceedingly brief and touch on salient features only. It will at least tend to show that the microscope, far from being the principal factor of psychiatric research, plays an entirely subordinate part.

PART II.*

THE CORRELATION OF SCIENCES IN THE INVESTIGATION OF MENTAL AND NERVOUS DISEASES.

CHAPTER V.

NORMAL PSYCHOLOGY AND PSYCHOPATHOLOGY.

The crowning glory of psychology in these days is its emancipation from metaphysics. Psychology has become a science. It has finally shown that the phenomena of the human mind are not vague and mysterious, but that their understanding is to be gained by methods of investigation such as are pursued in elucidating the phenomena of the world of life and matter generally; by means of the same general methods of investigations used in gaining knowledge of a distant star or a tiny organism. In gaining knowledge of the physical world, we make use of patiently observed phenomena, experiments and facts, and starting out with these we work out laws and hypotheses governing these facts. Modern psychology is proceeding in the same way with the phenomena of consciousness on the inductive—deductive basis. It is hard at work at the laboratory table, gathering facts, using instruments of precision, conducting experiments, assimilating similar work from kindred branches of sciences. In brief, modern psychology is one of observation and experimentation as against speculation on the

* In this part an attempt is made to plan out in a general way the main lines of research in mental and nervous diseases without much reference to the details of their application except by way of illustration. Since the Pathological Institute of the New York State Hospitals is largely based on this plan, we take the liberty of alluding to it in the text. This Institute was established in February, 1896. The departments of normal histology of the nervous system, of experimental pathology and hæmatology, although planned some time ago, are not yet in existence, but will be established, we hope, when more work will issue from the already active departments.

nature of the soul. It is building a foundation of facts to rest the superstructure of its doctrines and generalizations and laws of phenomena of the mind. All this has been brought about practically by the development of the science in this century. Weber and Fechner founded the domain of psychophysics. Fechner particularly invented new methods to study the intensity of sensations. He studied the laws governing the relations of the intensity of sensations to their stimuli. Much of his work in particular and of the school of the psychophysicists in general, following in Fechner's steps, though highly questionable, is still useful for its *negative* results. Hemholtz contributed much to psychology by his psycho-physiological studies on sensations. His magnificent intellect enabled him to apply the methods of not only one science, as physics, but to a whole group of sciences. For he was mathematician, anatomist, physiologist and a brilliant technician and worker with the microscope in unraveling the tangled fibres of the nervous system. Wundt introduced into psychology the most valuable of all methods in science, namely, the experimental method. The amount of work which Wundt has brought out from his Psychological Institute at Leipzig, most of which though giving small results, justly proclaim him as the great modern psychologist. In England, James Mill, John Stuart Mill, Bain, Spencer, Ward, Sully, Stout and others; in Italy, Mosso and others, have contributed their share to psychology. The names of Professor James and Professor Münsterberg are not to be omitted in this hasty sketch of the evolution of psychology into an exact science.

If the labors of general normal psychology have grown more scientific and practical, the work of psychopathology or abnormal psychology, embracing the psychological study of abnormal or pathological cases, has turned out to be of special importance not only from a theoretical standpoint in revealing the inner organization of mental life, but also from a purely practical standpoint, since *it has furnished the key to the understanding and even the treatment of functional nervous and mental diseases.* The results of psychopathology, some of which were obtained in our Institute, are brilliant in the extreme; they may be considered a treasure for medical science in general and for psychiatry in particular. No psychiatrist, no neurologist, can be efficient in his respective science without a knowledge of psychopathology. Functional neurosis, that stumbling block of the medical profession in general, and of the neurologist and psychiatrist in particular, can only be intelligently studied and successfully treated through the medium of psychopathology. Psychopathology is the *sine qua non* of the science of insanity, because insanity is a manifestation of more or less persistent pathological phenomena of consciousness, and psychopathology alone possesses the methods of investigating these pathological phenomena.

The work of the French school is particularly important, because of its remarkable contribution to the science of psychopathology. The French school with Ribot, Binet, and Janet at its head has been studying man's subconscious domain, a subject of the most profound importance, not only in that it touches at the heart of man's social attributes, but that the understanding of the nature of the subconscious is absolutely essential for any intelligent conception of the origin and course of mental maladies.

Finally the brilliant psychological and especially the psychopathological studies of Dr. Sidis *on dissociations in consciousness, linked with the parallel physiological dissociation of different realms of the brain, marks an important stage in the progress of psychology, and particularly psychopathology.* In Dr. Sidis' researches and studies of psychopathological cases, parts of the brain were dissociated from each other and the parallel psychic manifestations could be studied by themselves. Such experimental and clinical investigations help one not only to understand, but also to treat the similar isolated and split off fields of consciousness in different forms of nervous and mental diseases. Psychopathology helps to clear up hosts of difficulties that form almost insuperable obstacles in neurology and psychiatry.

Psychiatry is especially indebted to psychopathology, because it is only through the latter that psychiatry has any hopes of becoming a science relevant to its subject matter and have practical methods of treatment, based not on the rule of thumb, but on a solid scientific foundation. In fact we believe that psychopathology will ultimately replace the present would-be science of psychiatry. This sounds paradoxical, for psychiatry is generally considered to be the science of insanity. It claims the insane as its own. Unfortunately, psychiatry is a science in name only, it endeavors to be scientific, but fails in its attempt.

Psychiatry, in a certain sense, as hinted in a preceding chapter, is an overgrowth of the application of the methods of investigation of bodily diseases to those of the mind. Now it is absolutely hopeless to expect that methods applied to investigations of symptoms of somatic diseases are fit to apply to the investigation of mental maladies. These methods are absolutely incompetent, and even to a certain extent irrelevant.

The observation of the abnormal phenomena in insanity

relates to two groups of manifestations—the *somatic* and the *mental*. The *somatic* or *abnormal phenomena of the body*, including the abnormal manifestations of the lower parts of the nervous system, such as paralysis and the coarser and more obtrusive abnormal symptoms of the sense organs may be observed by the *clinical* methods of investigation. But in the study of *abnormal mental phenomena*, the disturbances of the higher forms of consciousness and the whole domain of psychomotor phenomena concomitant with dissociations of the higher spheres of the brain (where the nerve cells reach their highest complexity of organization in communities, clusters and constellations) lie beyond the scope of clinical methods of observation. These phenomena fall within the province of *pathological psychology* or *psychopathology*.

It should be more universally realized that there is a sharp dividing line between the efficacy of *clinical* and *psychopathological* methods of investigation in the study of insanity. This is an important matter, and one about which we should have clear and definite ideas in order not to make the mistake of believing that mental phenomena may be competently observed by clinical or somatic methods of investigation.

Psychiatry obeying the natural laws governing the general progress of science is still clinging to clinical investigation, in attempting to explore a territory beyond the scope of these methods. No fault is to be found with psychiatry for this state of affairs. If any criticism were justifiable, it should be regarded unfortunate that the normal psychologist has been so backward in taking up the study of pathological psychic phenomena, or psychopathology, and paving the way for the psychiatrist.

In discussing advance work in the study of abnormal organic life in the hospital, let us relegate *clinical* methods of investigation to their proper province, and not attempt the impossibility of stretching them over into the domain of abnormal mental phenomena, which can only be efficiently investigated by the methods of *psycho-pathology*. This same distinction between *clinical* and *psychopathological methods of investigation* deserves reflection in the study of *nervous diseases*. Psychiatry ought to embrace both fields of research in the study of insanity, the mental as well as the somatic; mamely, the investigation of the abnormal somatic phenomena and the pathological phenomena of the lower parts of the nervous system by clinical methods, and the investigation of the pathological mental phenomena by the methods of psychopathology.* It would seem appropriate, however, at present, to pin psychiatry down to the former domain where it belongs, and assign the latter to its proper sphere, pathological psychology or psychopathology. It is questionable if the psychopathologist would concede that even the pathological manifestations of the lower parts of the nervous system (and the effects of disease of these lower portions upon the higer ones), especially in functional diseases can be properly and completely investigated by the clinical methods of neuropathology and psychiatry. For all parts of the nervous system are too intimately interrelated in an organic whole to expect that the normal or pathological manifestations of these lower parts of the nervous system may be thoroughly comprehended by being isolated from the rest of the

*These methods and their application to the investigation of pathological mental manifestations are described by Dr. Sidis in a contribution from the Department of Psychology and Psychopathology now in press for a coming number of the ARCHIVES OF NEUROLOGY AND PSYCHOPATHOLOGY.

system and studied by themselves; or that the phenomena of any part of the system may be fully explained without a comprehensive knowledge of the phenomena of all other parts, the highest, the lowest, as well as the intermediate parts. Viewed in perspective the foreground of consciousness looms up beside the activity of the highest spheres of the brain composed of the most complex *constellations** of neurons while the vanishing point stretches away far down beside the activites of the lower and lowermost parts of the nervous system composed of mere elementary *groups*† of nerve cells. Thus psychopathology dealing with the pathological manifestations of consciousness *comprises a study of the phenomena of the lower parts of the nervous system* as well as of the higher portions and embraces especially the *interrelation between the two sets of phenomena in functional diseases.*

In the natural evolution of medicine, symptoms of bodily disease were worked out and differentiated first, then, after tedious halt behind all other departments of medicine, insanity was finally recognized as the symptom of abnormal conditions of the brain, and the methods of studying bodily symptoms were dragged over into the field of mental symptoms. Psychiatry in this stage of its evolution soon reached its limit of efficiency.

Psychiatry is an art and poses as a science. The science is only partially relevant to its subject. As an art it has done much. The simple recognition of the fact that insanity is a symptom of abnormal brain conditions, has overthrown the pernicious superstition of regarding the insane as possessed of devils. This alone has accomplished an enormous amount of good, and has resulted in an enlightened care of the material welfare of the patients

* Sidis, Psychology of Suggestion, Chap. XXI.
† Loc. Cit.

in our present hospitals for the insane. But we ought not mistake these advances in the art of psychiatry and think that they are scientific advances. In its wider sense, the art of psychiatry attends to the welfare of the insane as a dependent and helpless class upon the community.

The science of psychiatry deals with the whence and wherefore of mental diseases. The answer to these questions, however, psychiatry as a science, has largely failed to accomplish. A very simple and most elementary stage in the science of psychiatry was the recognition of the general fact that insanity is the symptom of pathological brain processes. This recognition rescued the insane from social revenge; at a later period from social indifference, and finally stimulated the active interference on the part of society for their welfare and humane treatment in the modern hospital of to-day. If all this progress in the art of psychiatry has been born of such an elementary and embryonic stage in its evolution as a science, how much more are we to expect in the prevention and cure of insanity in the future progress of this science? For as a science psychiatry is yet unborn, and can be brought into the world only by the aid of psychopathology. We now realize clearly the fact that writings from the standpoint of psychiatry as an art, must not pass for scientific disquisitions.

The psychiatrist on account of the incompetency of his methods is driven into the art field of psychiatry under the delusion that he is doing scientific work. Many in the field of psychiatry unconsciously bear out the criticism that scientific methods of investigating the symptoms of mental disease are merely an overgrowth of the methods used for investigating symptoms of bodily disease, by writing fine descriptions of the bodily ailments of the insane.

Fractures and dislocations of the insane are written up at length; the formation of their teeth, their palates, their hair, the occurrence of various complicating body diseases in great variety, such for instance as a fever, erysipelas, etc., are published in detail because the present psychiatric methods of investigation are better adapted to this sort of observations than for the investigation of insanity itself. Others find an opportunity for writing on medico-legal matters relating to the insane. Still others find distraction in the elaboration of statistics; others again in the field of therapeutics. Therapeutics, it is true, based on empirical knowledge of drugs has the recommendation of much common sense, because the knowledge gained thereby is founded on experience; but experience without reason is blind. The administration of drugs, particularly to the insane must rest on a rational basis, and this rational basis cannot come until we have an understanding and scientific explanation of insanity. When that time comes we may give fewer drugs, and perhaps in less quantities.

The pointing out of the unscientific character of this kind of literature may be unwelcome or unpleasant to many who are in daily touch with the insane. But if larger, broader and more inviting fields of real scientific investigation are indicated, no fault ought to be found with this presentation of the status of psychiatry. This should be reserved for those who criticise the work of the psychiatrist unintelligently, and who offer no new pathways for the old ones. It must not be understood that this pseudo scientific psychiatric literature, substituted for scientific work now possible by the advance of science, has no value. It has its peculiar interest; the only trouble with this kind of psychiatric literature is that its fields of investigation are so well burrowed and harrowed out that further work is only a loss of time and labor.

The investigation of the somatic phenomena in their relation to the pathological nervous processes and mental manifestations in the insane is of vital importance not only theoretically, but also practically, because from the body is derived the nourishment and the source of energy of the nervous system. It is, therefore, of the utmost consequence to understand the relation of disorders of the body to the interferences with the food supply of the nerve cells and the influence of toxic agents on these cells. The general somatic symptoms in insanity should be rewritten and revised as often as there are new discoveries and new theories in the progress of the pathology of bodily symptoms. Moreover, the bodily symptoms in each case in the hospital as an individual, irrespective of its class grouping or particular form of insanity, should receive detailed investigation because of the importance of the relation of the body to the brain in that the former provides the food supply, the source of energy of the nerve cell. It is, however, the fluctuations of neuron energy in their relation to the mental phenomena manifested that have to be principally studied.

We must be in possession of all the knowledge possible to gain about the bodily ailments of the insane and of those things that pertain to psychiatry as an art, but many of them are indicating a tendency towards stereotyped routine in psychiatric journal literature. Frankly speaking, gynæcological affairs, sprains, dislocations and fractures, the symptomatology of mere secondary complicating diseases of the body, such as fever, etc., are really rather round-about ways of getting at the scientific investigation and explanation of the *mental symptoms in insanity.*

Statistical work still leaves much to be done that is of the utmost value. Still, all things considered, much of the literature of psychiatry, even at the present day, is far from being scientifically satisfactory.

As an example of the tangle in which psychiatry finds itself at present, one may point to the hydra-headed classifications of mental diseases with fifty-four varieties of mania, and an equal number of melancholia, given in a standard compendium. There must be something wrong with a science that finds itself in such straits. Psychiatry has no methods appropriate for the investigation of abnormal mental phenomena; what wonder that it is impotent and cannot progress. Psychiatry must broaden out. As a science, psychiatry is absolutely dependent upon psychology and psychopathology and their correlative branches of science. Psychology and psychopathology have developed the real methods for gaining the facts, observing the phenomena and conducting the experiments that psychiatry needs. The great value then of pyschology and psychopathology is paramount in reviving the suspended animation of psychiatry.

It is unfortunate that both neurologists and psychiatrists have a tendency to view psychology as so much metaphysics, or to sum up the whole practical utility of normal psychology and psychopathology with the word hypnotism, as though the sum total of the immense value of psychological and psychopathological methods of investigation and practical lessons of their teachings are bound to be centered about the phenomena of hypnosis. If there is to be any ultimate, tangible and firm basis for the understanding of mental diseases, and a consequent rational treatment and classification of them, it is surely to come as a result of the use of the methods of psychology and psychopathology. Space forbids any more than an allusion to the great value of understanding the psychic phenomena of the normal individual by studying the disordered psychic phenomena in abnormal individuals. Scientific researches of normal mental and nervous processes seldom have their full value without the observation and experiment of pathological cases, nature's experiments. In many forms of insanity, nature is performing experiments, more ingenious and valuable for study than the psychologist, restricted to the study of the phenomena of the normal consciousness, could ever devise. Normal psychology has much to learn and in fact can itself not be firmly established without a previous thorough exploration of the domain of pathological psychology.

In one instance, at least, under the direction of Kraepelin at Heidelberg, have the results of studies in pathological psychology been most satisfactory in clearing away some of the mystery surrounding the origin of mental diseases. The extensive experiments at this school on the subject of fatigue of the nervous system have already stimulated a more exact and broader view of the study of the symptoms of insanity. But even this school has failed to study mental diseases directly at their fountain-head; it is only through such a work that we can get an insight into the nature of mental aberrations. The Department of Psychology and Psychopathology at the Institute devotes its time mostly to the study of pathological cases.

It will not be inappropriate here to make a mere allusion to three prominent cases in which the Department has not only cleared up much of the explanation of the symptoms but worked out of the laws of the disease, the methods of cure, and applied them successfully. Psychopathology yielded definite tangible results of the highest value.

The first case was from the Binghamton State Hospital, and was studied in conjunction with Dr. William A. White. The case presented limitation of the field of vision, accompanied by occasional attacks of delirium and many other phenomena of mental dissociation. The case was closely studied experimentally; very important phenomena were elicited and a general method for the investigation and cure of similar cases discovered.

The second case was sent to the Institute through the courtesy of Professor B. Sachs, of New York city. It was one of functional hemi-anæsthesia and ataxia complicated with organic disorders. Investigation controlled and eliminated the functional disorders, which were of long standing, and had previously resisted all attempts at improvement.

The third case, known under the name of total amnesia and "double consciousness," yielded theoretical and practical discoveries of the most brilliant nature to science in general and psychology in particular. From the investigation of this case were deduced laws guiding treatment for future cases, which, up to the time of these researches, were left to the care of Providence as lying beyond the ken of human knowledge.

All of these cases were quite beyond the use of drugs, and far beyond investigation by any of the methods which neurology and psychiatry make use of, and in both cases the treatment based on theoretical studies in psychopathology was crowned with complete success.

This Department also works in the lines of *cellular psychopathology, correlating the different psychomotor* *manifestations with the varied affections of the neuron and fluctuations in neuron energy.* This is an attempt, and the first of its kind, to bring into one comprehensive scheme and embrace in one formula *expressed in terms of the fluctuations in neuron energy with the concomitant psychomotor manifestations* the infinite number of bewildering phenomena met with in nervous and mental diseases.* Along with it the laws and principles of inter-relation of the neurons are worked out; these, we hope in due time may lead to some important laws forming the scientific basis of pathology in general, and of pathology of the nervous system in particular.

This same department in connection with that of experimental pathology and physiological chemistry is also undertaking work in comparative psychopathology. The simulacra of diseases like catalepsy, paralysis agitans or epilepsy, for instance, we are endeavoring to induce artificially in animals. The manifestations are closely studied and experimented upon, and are then correlated with nervous diseases in men that give like symptoms under the same conditions of experimentation.

This mere fleeting glimpse of the relations of psychopathology to psychiatry does not, however, regard many other great side avenues in other departments of abnormal mental and nervous life. In the prison, the reformatory, the hospital for the epileptic, in the institutions for the feeble-minded and idiots and for the general delinquent and defective mental classes psychopathology has a great field to reap. Its lines of research are the most prominent and valuable in the institutions furnishing the meeting-ground for the criminal and the victim of insanity—the

* Vide "Neuron Energy and its Psychomotor Manifestations." ARCHIVES OF NEUROLOGY AND PSYCHOPATHOLOGY, Jan., 1898.

hospital for the criminal insane. *In fact the so-called criminal anthropology is largely a domain of psychopathology*, only the physical data and measurements properly fall within the field of anthropology.

To strengthen the importance of the wider application of psychopathology in medicine by enumerating the diseases whose investigation demands its services is unnecessary since this would comprise nearly the whole great list of mental and nervous diseases. While the most brilliant domain of psychopathology is in the functional diseases of the higher realms* of the nervous system including neurasthenia, hysteria, epilepsy, etc., the investigation of the more focal or localized diseases of the nervous system and nervous diseases generally has great gains to score through the aid of pathological psychology. In nervous diseases the absence of psychopathological investigation has enforced an unfortunate negligence of the mental phenomena in these diseases. In the study of lesions of the "silent"—although to psychopathology eloquently silent—regions of the brain, especially the frontal lobes, neurological methods have made a frank confession of their defeat. In the whole group of apraxias, aphasias, amnesias and the like are inviting arenas for psychopathology. The vista of psychopathology stretches out far and wide. The science will illuminate the darkest recesses of the nervous system above all the brain.

Enough has been said to insist upon the maintenance of a Department of Psychology and Psychopathology at the scientific Institute of the New York State Hospitals, as the one the most closely affiliated with, and in fact of paramount importance in the study of insanity.

* Vide Psychopathic Waking and Sleeping States (Chart II) in "Neuron Energy," ARCHIVES, Jan., '98.

This department is provided with a reasonable outfit of instruments. It is provided with sphymographs, cardiographs, pneumographs, chronographs, ergographs, reaction-timers, etc. Some of these instruments have been made to order; others, bought in Europe. In fact, the equipping of the Department of Psychology and Psychopathology takes an amount of time which seems unintelligible to those who might expect work to come forth from an Institute of this kind with undue haste. The apparatus of this department is as yet rather meagre, and it serves only its most fundamental requirements. In the course of time, other instruments will have to be added as the department and its work will grow and develop. It cannot develop all at once and spring forth into full activity, like Minerva from the head of Jupiter. It has been thought unwise, therefore, to add apparatus to the equipment of the department beyond what is absolutely indispensable for the carrying on of the work on hand. The same is to be said of every other department in this Institute.

Within the brief space of the foundation of this department its work has grown so extensive, the problems on hand are so numerous, that an increase in its working force is absolutely essential. Without an assistant the chief of this department must lose the opportunity of taking up works of the utmost value. Psychology and psychopathology has been the central inspiration of all of the branches of research of this Institute for they have infused into the several avenues of work a spirit of philosophy, the soul of progress in any science. The department of Normal Psychology and Psychopathology is under the charge of Boris Sidis, M. A., Ph.D., (Harvard).

Chapter VI.

NORMAL HISTOLOGY OF THE NERVOUS SYSTEM.

The story of the evolution of our knowledge of the structure of the human nervous system is full of interest, if not fascination, but we can only touch upon it here in the baldest outline, sufficiently to appreciate its status at the present day.

The first and very meagre chapter containing any real insight into the marvels of the structure of the nervous system, begins with Descartes. The keenness of perception of this remarkable man enabled him long before the microscope had been invented, to portray the structure of the nerve fibres, both in diagrams and in text. He considered them as minute tubules which conveyed the animal spirits from the brain to the muscles. If we substitute for the word animal spirits the modern phrase nervous impulse, Descartes in his idea of the nerve fibres was not so very far behind our conception of this structure at the present day.

After a lapse of some three hundred years, in the early part of this century, the microscope demonstrated that the nerve fibre was not hollow, but contained a solid core, or axis. A little later in the early thirties, investigators discovered that the brain not only contained untold numbers of these nerve tubules with the solid core, but myriads and myriads of tiny lumps of protoplasm, the nerve cells.

At that day, workers in the field of the microscopical anatomy of the brain were utterly unable to solve the riddle of the relationship of the cells on the one hand and the fibres on the other. No one knew where the fibres came from, or where they ended, nor was any one able to make out the least connection of the fibres among themselves. The whole nervous system was an inextricable snarl of an infinite number of fibres and nerve cells, hopelessly tangled and mixed up together. It was, therefore, impossible to obtain any idea as to how this greatest marvel of creation—the human brain—did its work. At this period, the microscope was in a crude condition, as compared with the powerful instrument of investigation of modern times. For to-day the construction of lenses has so advanced and their magnifying power is so great that a unit of measurement for the minute anatomist of to-day working with the microscope is only $\frac{1}{25000}$ of an inch long.

In the early thirties the brain histologist or minute anatomist had to study his material in fresh condition. He had no methods of preservation; nor did he enjoy the advantages of being able to cut thin, diaphanous slices from the brain to view under the microscope. To-day we have the whole armamentarium of the chemist to preserve the brain in a hundred different ways, which gives as many variations of methods of study. We have apparatus for cutting thin sections of the nervous system, so delicately contrived that twenty thousand of these sections piled on top of each other would not be an inch high. Moreover, to-day one has at hand a hundred aniline dyes and other colors with which to stain these sections, color and pick out selectively elements of the nervous system in the sections under the microscope so as to suit his particular purpose.

The whole record of progress in the structure of the brain invariably goes hand in hand with a similar record of improvements in the microscope and other apparatus and also in technical methods of investigation.

During the forties and fifties, investigators began to shed some light on the obscurity of the structure of the nervous system by discovering one exceedingly important fact, namely, that the cells and fibres were not independent of each other, but that the fibre was a prolongation of the cell, an outgrowth of its body. This at least cleared up the question as to the origin of the fibre, and physiologists derived comfort from this fact, in that they had a reasonable explanation of how, in a fundamental fashion, the nervous system operated. The nerve cell, so to speak, was the headquarters of nervous operations, and its enormously long outstretched arm in the form of a fibre, was a device to carry the impulse to some distant part. This important fact as to the connection of nerve fibre and nerve cell did not contribute as much toward advancing knowledge of the nervous system as might have been expected. The connection of the nerve fibre and nerve cell was only witnessed in the very simplest parts of the nervous system, and not in its more complex and most highly developed parts of the brain itself. Besides this, while the early investigators were sure that the nerve fibre came out of the nerve cell, they were still ignorant of the course and termination of the fibre. They saw the origin of one end of the fibre only, the part which sprang from the cell.

Thus until fifteen or twenty years ago the structure of the nervous system was still a riddle and a puzzle. The whole nervous system was an inextricable maze of an entangled net-work and its unraveling seemed impossible. It was hopeless confusion to attempt to follow out the pathway of a single nervous impulse in this labyrinthic net-work. Within the past ten or fifteen years the obscurity that enshrouded the nervous system was replaced by a clear and definite insight, that is almost startling. In 1873 a distinguished Italian investigator discovered a method which revolutionized our whole knowledge of the structure of the nervous system and opened boundless fields of research in manifold directions. From the results of this method of investigation, we have a final solution of the structure of the nerve cell, the nerve fibre and their connections.

The nerve cell is like a tiny octopus. Like this animal it has a body whereby it attends to the process of digestion and assimilation. In this body, a food supply from the blood vessels is elaborated into materials which enable the cell to do its work. Like the octopus, too, from one end of the body of the nerve cell springs out a multitude of branching arms or tentacles. From another part of the cell body arises an arm different from the shorter arms or tentacles. This arm is of exceedingly great length, and passes away from the body to distances hundreds and thousands of times the diameter of the cell itself. The outstretched arms of the nerve cell octopus—the nerve fibre—may pass to the outer parts of the body, where they receive messages from the eye or ear, or other sense organs. The long arm passes out to other parts of the nervous system, to transmit impulses from one part of the nervous system to another. These octopus like nerve cells are arranged in *groups*, *systems*, *clusters*, *communities* and *constellations** of exceeding complexity.

A given nerve cell octopus passes its long outstretched arm so as to touch the tentacles or shorter arms of a second octopus. The second one, in turn, passes its long arm to the tentacles of the third and so on through an infinite set of combinations which have their highest

* Sidis, Psychology of Suggestion, Ch. XXI.

complexity of arrangement in the highest spheres of our brain, which are the last parts to develop, both in the evolution of species as well as the individual, and which are ever unstable and prone to disintegrate by reason of the process of retraction of the nerve cells.

In the lower parts of the nervous system retraction and the corresponding dissociation of the functioning groups of nerve cells is less liable to occur under the influence of pathogenic agencies. For here the functions are phylogenetically older and tend to approach more or less a stereotyped nature. Since the stability of organization of the different parts of the nervous system depends on the frequency of the impulses transmitted through the group of neurons, the lower parts of the nervous system are more firmly united than are the highest spheres of the brain.*

The most interesting feature of this latter-day conception of the make-up of the nervous system, is that the nerve cell, like the octopus, possesses power of movement over its tentacles.† Consider, for a moment, what happens when the nerve cell retracts its tentacles. The message can be no longer transmitted. The nerve cell has thrown itself out of the circuit of the long arms of its fellow-associates in a given group or community; they are no longer in contact with the retracted tentacle. But we should conceive that as a rule whole groups, communities, clusters

* This was written before Apathy's view of the concrescence of neurons came to our attention. We were thus, in a measure, prepared *a priori* to accept his views not for the whole nervous system but its lower and phylogenetically oldest portions.

† From a study of the identity of differentiation which the general structure of the neuron undergoes in the neuraxone in the form of long parallel filaments incorporated with distinct microsomes with analogous modifications of the cyto-reticulum in other somatic cells (muscle cell, ciliated cell, leucocyte, chromatophores, etc.) subservient to motility, my own observations incline me to believe that the axone may be the retractile and expansive structure of the neuron as well as the dendrons or gemmules.

and constellations of nerve cells functionally correlated retract *en masse* rather than individual cells. Cells cannot work as isolated individuals in the higher parts of the nervous system; they are invariably members of assemblages which have been physiologically linked together by education, use and function. There may be partial retraction of the individual members of one functionally linked assemblage of neurons from another assemblage, but in the phenomenon of retraction we are to picture it occurring in a mass of nerve cells belonging to some particular assemblage and occurring more or less simultaneously.

A message can no longer be delivered and transmitted from one part of the nervous system to another, if a mass of these nerve cells break the circuit by retracting their arms. This is the secret of many a puzzle and mystery enveloping a very great mass of psychomotor manifestations of the human nervous system. The object which the nerve cell apparently has in view in retracting its arms is to avoid overwork, and withdraw itself from hurtful stimuli. Retraction of the arms of the nerve cell is apparently a signal of exhaustion of the dynamic energy of the neuron.

Retraction is a remarkable adaptation of the higher order of neuron aggregates to elude stimuli (energy liberating impulses) which increasing in quantity or degree would otherwise draught off deeper and deeper levels of static neuron energy. And expenditure of static neuron energy is a process marking the passage of the psychomotor manifestations from the physiological domain to the realm of disease. In other words retraction of the neuron may be regarded as an adaptation whereby increased resistance is interposed to energy liberating impulses which have exhausted the high potential energy stored in the neuron for the activities of the physiological waking states.

Neuron aggregates are united to each other by training, by function. The more simple the aggregates and the more frequently they functionate together the more stable is the union. The stability of the functional association is established by routine use, by habit. On the other hand the more complex are the neuron aggregates, that is the greater variety and permutations of their association with sub-aggregates, the less stable is the association. Instability of neuron aggregations reaches its *maximum* in the highest orders of constellations, for here there is but little or no permanency of the functional interaction—there is no routine beaten track, no set channels of the associations in the highest order of constellations. In a simple reflex arc the external stimuli are of a uniform kind and always proceed in the same pathway. In the highest constellations of neurons the stimuli come through a great variety of avenues. At one instant the impulse wells up through some particular avenue, at another instant the stimuli preponderate in another channel. The result is a continual flux in the functional association of the higher constellations. The functional association is subject to continual mutability, to continual forming and unforming of the associations with other neuron aggregates. This is in fact the physiological parallel of the swell and play of the human mind, the infinite variety of thought and reasoning. Association and dissociation of the higher orders of neuron aggregates may be conceived as continually taking place in *normal* mental life concomitant with the activities of the higher realms of consciousness. As Sidis explains it "under the action of the slightest external or internal stimuli unstable systems* or constellations lose their equilibrium, dissolve and form new systems or enter into combination with other constellations. On the psychical side we have the continuous fluctuation of the content of attention. *The characteristic trait of the highest type of psychophysical life under the ordinary stimuli of the environment is a continuous process of association and dissociation of constellations.*"

Association and *dissociation* of neuron aggregates then form the physiological parallel of normal mental life. *Retraction* and *expansion* of neuron aggregates form the corresponding physiological parallel of abnormal mental life. In accordance with the laws of stability of neuron aggregations the highest and last trained constellations in the psychophysiological evolution offer the least resistance to stimuli or agencies which liberate neuron energy. If the stimulus becomes intense, or what amounts to the same thing, is persistent although of mild intensity, the most unstable constellations lose their dynamic energy first. After the dynamic energy is exhausted retraction occurs and the stimulus is evaded. Concomitantly with the retraction of the least stable constellations a sphere of consciousness is split off from the whole. If the stimulus increases still farther the retraction progresses to deeper and deeper levels in the organization of the nervous system. Clusters of neurons offering less resistance in their functional aggregation than the communities, become retracted and fall asunder. With an increase of the stimulus communities undergo dissociation among themselves and so on down to neuron aggregates which by

* By means of association fibres neuron aggregates are built up from simple to complex orders. Simple and through function firmly interwoven groups are organized into systems by association fibres. Systems are organized into communities, communities into clusters, clusters into constellations.

reason of stereotyped functional interaction are organically united. In these lowest neuron aggregates the adaptation of retraction and expansion is superfluous and might even be inimical to life.

This retraction and expansion of the arm of the nerve cell, in groups, systems and communities of brain cells, drawing it in or out of the circuit of transmission of nervous impulse, is the final unveiling of the secret of a whole host of mental phenomena which hitherto have seemed mysterious to the last degree. These attributes of extension and expansion of the nerve cell cannot fail to attract even those with the most casual interest in the operations and development of the human mind, and holds one spellbound in the vast flood of light shed upon the explanation of insanity. Mysterious cases, for instance, of individuals who sometimes from a blow upon the head or other causes, wake up and find their past lives a blank, and who virtually begin to live their lives over again as it were, in a new world, such as a case recounted in Dr. Sidis' book "The Psychology of Suggestion" may serve as a fair example. Such cases receive their only explanation in retraction and expansion of the tentacles of the nerve cell octopus, *dissociating functioning associations of cells.*

The phenomena of hypnotism, hysteria, and of the whole great important groups of *psychopathic functional diseases* are to be explained in the same way.* Some of the violent manifestations of insanity seem to be due to the retraction of the highest constellations of nerve cells that dominate and control the lower parts of our nervous system. The lower centres being dissociated from the control of the higher ones, give rise to the phenomena found in some forms of mania (psychopathic). Discrim-

* The topic is further elaborated in the Principles of Psychopathology, a work recently completed by Dr. Sidis.

ination as to significant and insignificant stimuli is cast aside, so the maniac is prone to respond to any passing zephyr of stimulus with a storm of excitement. His subconsciousness lacks the normal control and is most prominently in the foreground.

The phenomenon of retraction of the neurons is also, I most firmly believe, the explanation of the cardinal symptoms of epilepsy in the manifestations of the fit. Here the retraction of the constellations and clusters in the higher parts (association centres of Flechsig), from a given stimulus is very sudden; the lower portions of the brain (sensory spheres of Flechsig, particulary tacto-motor zone) being suddenly loosened and dissociated from the inhibition and control of the higher portions, the energy of the neurons of these lower portions of the cortex is suddenly liberated with the corresponding psycho-motor phenomena.

Every one is familiar with those forms of insanity in which the patient seems oblivious to his outside environment, shown in some forms of melancholia (psychopathic). There are again instances where the whole foreground of consciousness has been *partially* split off by a retraction of the nerve cells constituting the higher spheres of the brain. A cleft lies between them and the rest of the nervous system, caused by this phenomena of retraction. Depending upon the quantitative degree of retraction between various assemblages of neurons in the brain some forms of psychopathic mania or melancholia might result. Thus we see that one part or another of the brain may be dissociated from the rest, and naturally the parallel manifestations of the mind are thrown out of gear.

This hasty sketch of the department devoted to the

anatomy of the nervous system, perhaps, shows best of all a faint glimpse of the directions we are striving in to contribute something toward clearing up the explanation of insanity. These introductory paragraphs ought also to show how important this department is for the investigation of insanity.

I should not, however, be guilty of conveying the impression that merely because the anatomist has discovered these wonderful facts about the shape of the nerve cell and its connections or that some evidence from my own researches tends to prove the phenomena of retraction, that the study of mental phenomena is superfluous. The anatomist, the chemist cannot possibly disclose *thought*, *consciousness* from the material phenomena with which they respectively deal. The work of the psychologist and especially of the psychopathologist attains its highest importance when the physiological processes concomitant with the mental phenomena studied are constantly kept in view. The dynamic theory of cellular life and the theory of neuron retraction in fact can be most safely worked out from the psychopathological standpoint in conjunction with the study of general physiology. The anatomist or the chemist do not have *consciousness* for their material. Thought is not a *product* of nerve cell activity in the same sense as bile is a product of the liver. The brain does not secrete thought, as the kidneys secrete urine; thought is not a material thing; it can neither be weighed nor measured. A sensation of color, for instance, as experienced by the eye, has no material existence in the physical world. We can only speak of the phenomena of consciousness as running parallel or being concomitant with the metabolism of the nerve cell, lest we make of consciousness a material body.

To the psychologist belongs the study of psychophysiological life; the details of structure fall within the sphere of the anatomist. The object of reverting back to the department of psychology and psychopathology is briefly to point out the incongruity of setting forth the claims of any of these departments of the Institute investigating insanities as distinct, isolated methods of research. They must all be linked together and work hand in hand. A concrete example of this is the apportionment and yet linking together of the work in the departments of psychology and normal anatomy of the nervous system. The psychologist, for instance, studies the manifestations concomitant with the physiological process of retraction of the tentacles of the nerve cell octopus. Working conjointly, the psychologist and the anatomist show, in an ideally scientific way, the stages of the *parallelism* of the physical process in the nerve cell and the corresponding psychic phenomena.

In the section devoted to the status of the science of pathology in investigating the nervous system, the same feature crops out again. In the abnormal anatomy of the nervous system as well as in the normal anatomy in the necessity for correlated work with psychological and psychopathological investigation is still more evident.

The anatomist, however, is not by any manner of means in a position to write the last words about the structure and architecture of the human nervous system. This goal will not be attained for many years to come. He has only been able thus far to straighten out the intricate structure and connections of the comparatively elementary chains and series of the octopus-like nerve cells in the lower and simpler parts of the nervous system. The unravelling of the connections and associations of nerve cells in the highest parts of the nervous system, where the cells are evolved in enormous complexity of connections in the form of constellations, hardly has been begun. By studying the developing infant, however, and patiently working at the brain of the growing child, we hope to attain in the future our best light upon this obscure domain of the anatomist.

Professor Flechsig has, however, after twenty years of work, formulated a plan of the brain which, it seems to me, is the key for a final solution of the intricacies of higher brain architecture. This plan was studied out in the brains of human embryos, children at birth and growing infants, where the different parts of the nervous system can be identified because they make their appearance in a progressive series from the simple, fundamental and phylogenetically oldest parts to the more complex, highly organized and most recently evolved portions.

In accordance with this plan of Flechsig, but a small portion of the brain cortex—only one-third—comes in contact with the outside world through the chains and series of octopus-like nerve cells connecting the sense organs, while the great mass of the brain cortex—the remaining two-thirds—has no direct connection with the outer world, but connects and associates the scattered brain areas connected with the sense organs or muscles.

This division of the brain into these two parts—the smaller portion known as the sensory spheres and the larger the association centres—gives a wonderfully clear view into many forms of insanity if we take into account the concomitant psychomotor phenomena produced by different degrees of retraction of these parts, but especially by retractions occurring in the association centres themselves by retractions of communities, clusters and constellations of nerve cells.

The sensory spheres are scattered about in the cortical grey matter. A patch at the hind end of the brain is the sensory sphere for vision, another corresponding to the sensory sphere for sound is situated near the apex of the temporal lobe. Similarly olfactory, gustatory and tacto-motor sensory spheres are located in other parts of the cortex. Between the sensory spheres are interpolated the association centres. The more fundamental portions of the association centres operate to render possible a simple order of recognition of the impressions received in the sensory spheres by associating them together. In the higher regions of the association centres a still more complex order of recognition of sensory and motor impressions is possible. Finally the constellations of nerve cells probably located in the frontal lobes afford a basis for the highest forms of synthesis of consciousness. *This is the association centre of association centres.*

It is in these association centres and in their connections with the sensory spheres that the phenomena of retraction of the nerve cell plays such an important part. One can well conceive the chaotic condition of ideas, or imperfect power of recognition, and a host of other abnormal mental phenomena, when retractions occurring in the groups, communities, clusters and complex constellations of nerve cells split off the association centres, from each other or from the sensory spheres, and *produce corresponding dissociations in consciousness.* In the lower animals the association centres grow smaller and smaller, and finally, say for instance, in the lower mammals, the sensory spheres lie contiguous with hardly any vestige of the association centres between them.

For the study of insanity, the understanding of the structure of these higher spheres of the nervous system is of the most vital importance. It is the instability of these highest parts of the nervous system which is the essence of the whole question of insanity. Hence, when we consider this aspect of the value of the department of normal histology of the nervous system, we find that its offices are absolutely indispensable.

With the exception of the discovery of the neuron theory, Sidis' psychophysiological theory of association and dissociation, the theory of the retraction and expansion of the neurons, the theory of neuron energy fluctuation, and Flechsig's plan of the association centres and sensory spheres of the brain are the greatest discoveries which have ever been put forth in the history of our knowledge of the nervous system. The effect of the application of these great hypotheses (for observations* at present in my own belief, at least, are increasing their validity) will indeed be revolutionary in the domain of mental and nervous diseases.

One standpoint in this chapter I trust is clear, and that is, we thoroughly understand that normal histology of the nervous system should not be confined to a study of the mere static side of mental and nervous life but should go hand in hand with a study of its dynamics. We cannot

* Apathy's theory of the concrescences of the neurons in the lowest parts of the nervous system may be perfectly tenable. But we should remember that the stereotyped function existing through eons of time in these lowest parts of the nervous system presupposes a fixed relation of the neurons to each other. In the evolution of the higher centres however, such as the association centres and probably the sensory spheres, the individual neurons have become independent anatomically and the impulse is transmitted by physiological contact.

Retraction does not take place in the lowest parts of the nervous system, but must be postulated for the phenomena of the highest portions of the brain. Apathy's theory, in my judgment, should not create distrust in the neuron theory; his theory does not apply to the whole nervous system, but to its lowermost parts, such as pertain to the most automatic and vegetative functions. The homologue of the lowest parts of the human nervous system is found in the leech and other invertebrates that Apathy has studied.

grasp the laws governing the dynamics of life by the study of morphology. One cannot see physiological processes in cut and dried sections through the microscope. Life phenomena are manifestations of energy. To understand the dynamic side of life phenomena one must use the principles of general physiology. For this science studies the real internal causes of the activities of living matter in energy and the laws of the equivalence of cause and effect in the phenomena of life in the liberation and restitution cycles of energy. The operations of mind however, are not modes of motion although running parallel with them. Life and matter fall within the monistic principle of energy, but mind is something apart and cannot be explained by the doctrine of energy. Physiology stands far above anatomy in its philosophy. Psychology occupies a still higher plane, for in addition to the knowledge of both that of consciousness is required.

Although realizing the great necessity of establishing the department of Normal Histology, I have not, in view of the considerable sum already expended in organizing and developing this Institute, had the temerity to ask for further expenditure in obtaining a salary for the associate in this branch until some tangible results in scientific work have been brought forth. I would now, however, *make claims for the necessity of this branch of work*, so that within the future, perhaps the ensuing year, a recommendation for its establishment may seem reasonable and fit.

It is appropriate to intimate that the associate of this line of research should pursue his studies of the normal histology of the nervous system, only after a very thorough antecedent study of the minute anatomy of all other parts of the body in order that he may be sure to have the light of analogy of the neuron with other cells of the body constantly in mind.

Chapter VII.

COMPARATIVE NEUROLOGY.

The value of the comparative study of the nervous system in both health and disease, has been hinted at in the argument for the practical value of the department of cellular biology in the scientific study of insanity. Man's nervous system is a recapitulation of the progression of development of the nervous system in animals. This recapitulation of the nervous system embracing its evolution throughout the whole animal kingdom is too complex to be understood without going back to the prologue in the history of the development in the lowest animals that possess nervous organs.

Apparently the first nucleus of a nervous system is found in the fresh water hydra. This creature can expand and retract a portion of its substance by a very simple mechanism, which is the combination of both the nervous and muscular systems. This animal appreciates stimuli from the external environment by means of a most elementary sensory apparatus, the fore-shadow of the nervous system in higher animals, and reacts by means of a primitive muscular mechanism. These two sets of mechanisms are not differentiated as in the higher animals into two distinct organizations, but are so alike and undifferentiated that it is difficult to distinguish the one from the other.

In a somewhat higher form of development, as in an ascidian, the motor and nervous systems have become differentiated. This creature has an outer tunic, an inner digestive coat and a muscular sac lying between the two. The nervous apparatus is exceedingly simple. It is merely a chain composed of very few nerve cells, one end of which touches the outside tunic, and the other end the muscular coat. When stimuli from the external environment are conveyed to the tunic, the creature, by means of this nervous system, transmits the impulses to the muscular bag, and responds by muscular movements to these stimuli. The very simple nervous system in this creature is the fundamental basis for the building up of the nervous system in the higher animals. This tiny arc of nerve cells passing between the muscle and the skin in the ascidian is the starting point which nature builds upon in evolving the wonderfully complex nervous apparatus in higher animals and in man himself. Roughly speaking, the difference between man's nervous system and that of the ascidian is not in any essential distinction in the shape and constitution of the nerve cell, but in the fact that man possesses numerically millions and millions more, in infinitely complex adjustment, of these tiny nerve cell arcs found in the ascidian.

Passing upward in the scale of evolution from the ascidian, as more and more of these nerve cell arcs make their appearance, and are evolved into increasingly complex adjustment to each other, the animal gains more and more highly developed functions. In the lowest forms of animal life possessing the nervous system, the nerve cells are arranged in simple *chains or series*,* as the evolution of the animal grows more complex, the simple series make a greater variety of combinations with each other, so that they become gathered together into *groups*.* As the scale of evolution becomes still higher, groups of nerve cells make increasingly complex adjustments in the form of *clusters*.* In still higher forms of animal life, the adjustment of clusters

*See Sidis " Psychology of Suggestion, Chap. XXI.

of nerve cells become complicated into *communities.** In man we find all the evolutionary series compounded into one complex whole. The elementary form of the nervous system in the lower animal represented in a simple *chain* or *series* of nerve cells, is present in the lower and more fundamental parts of his nervous system, such as the sympathetic. The more complex forms are built up into *groups*, *clusters*, *communities*, and ultimately in the highest parts of man's brain, the *communities* are gathered together in such a variety of combinations as to form an infinite number of highly complex *constellations.**

In building up this plan of the nervous system from the lowest to the highest creatures, nature makes no sudden strides or leaps. It is a steady progression of piling up the simple series of nerve cells, such as found in the ascidian, in increasing numbers and complexity of combination until we reach the form of constellations in the highest portion of man's brain. His intellectual attainments, his highest form of consciousness, his self-control and dominance of the lower parts of his nervous system run parallel with the activities of these constellations.

Comparative anatomy of the nervous system is invaluable as a method of going back through past ages, and of witnessing how man's nervous system has been built up from the simple to the complex. All the chapters in the history of brain evolution are to come from the researches of comparative neurology. We must not expect to comprehend the architecture and phenomena of man's nervous system by considering it as something apart from the nervous system of the creatures whence he is derived. Nature did not make man's nervous system by a special *fiat*, nor in evolving it did she consider him to be any more

* See Sidis "Psychology of Suggestion," Chap. XXI.

or less than the final member of a continuous series in the progression of the evolution of life forms.

Man is to be looked upon as a creature of the past. For nature in the evolution of the nervous system has built man on the same fundamental plan with that of an ascidian. Man's nervous system is a magnificent organization, but in plan of structure it is the same in the ape, the dog or even the earth worm.

Comparative anatomy of the nervous system has often given us the most striking answers to complicated questions in man's brain. For instance, when certain animals leave their aquatic habitat and spend the rest of their existence leading a terrestrial life, special sense-organs become useless and disappear during the terrestrial life. The following out of the changes of the brain, incident to the loss of these sense-organs has thrown most important light upon some of the complicated questions of the nerves in man's brain. The enfeebled development of eyesight in the mole, and the deficient development of the portions of the brain concerned with its visual impressions have helped us in understanding the central mechanism of vision in man's brain. The enormous development of the sense of smell and of the parts of the brain devoted to the reception of olfactory impressions in the lower animals has been of much service in contributing to the knowledge of the structure of the parts of man's brain connected with his delicate but uncomprehensive sense of smell. In fact, in the study of man's brain, we are constantly driven back into the past when it was in a simpler form, in order to understand its mechanism and operations.

Comparative neurology is of value, not only in helping us to understand the architecture of the nervous system, *but it is also destined to be of great importance in imparting knowledge of the organization of the nerve cell as an individual, through the study of comparative cytology of the nerve cell.* An individual nerve cell, a single one of the myriads and myriads composing man's brain is a microcosm taken by itself. We are far from knowing, aside from the problem of how nerve cells are connected with each other in the brain, how they work as individuals, how they live and die and pass through their whole life history. If we had the most perfect knowledge of all the combinations, adjustments and associations of the countless hosts of nerve cells in the brain, in short a perfect knowledge of the architecture, it would be of comparatively little value in the study of insanity, unless we understood the *nerve cell as an individual.* No one could build a bridge, even with the most perfect and detailed working plans, without knowing the constitution of the building materials. So it is with the nervous system. We may know much as to its architecture, and in fact are actually daily gaining more and more of this kind of knowledge by a great variety of methods, but we know comparatively little of the working units of the nervous system, the nerve cells.

The internal constitution of the nerve cells is the most pressing question of the day in the study of insanity. The all-important question is how the nerve cell works as an individual, how it conducts nervous impulses, how it assimilates food, and the mechanism of elaboration of energy from the crude food supply which the nerve cell obtains from the blood vessels. If there be one all-important question in the production of insanity, it relates to the *balance between food supply of the nerve cells* and the *work performed or withdrawal of nervous energy.* This is a practical question, because everyone knows that if more energy is drawn off from the nerve cell than can be produced from its food supply, the result is bankruptcy of the nervous system. Anyone may see this in his daily walks of life in the man who overworks and overfatigues his nervous system. We see this debit balance in the energy of the nervous system everywhere about us in the endeavor to cheat time in the pressure of hurry and haste in the activity of large cities. People expend more energy from their nervous system than they supply through food and rest. Yet such a vitally important question as to the details of the cycles of expended energy of the nerve cell, with relation to food supply, is almost unknown. Here again we must have recourse to the aid of the comparative neurologist, but above all to the science of general physiology. We must ask him to tell us the internal structure and constitution of the nerve cells in the lower animals, because here the problem may be studied under its simplest condition. We ask him to make experiments, and to select some favorable animal to illustrate the changes of fatigue in the nerve cell, to tell us what happens when the nerve cell is deprived of its food supply, to recount to us the changes in the constitution of the nerve cell, when it is called to expend more energy than it receives in nourishment. Such questions as these are of the utmost importance.

As a concrete illustration of experimental work in comparative neurology I might mention an off-hand example in some work which we had undertaken some three years ago in the electric torpedo to determine what happened in the nerve cell when overfatigued. Two torpedoes were placed side by side. One was irritated at regular intervals with a sharp instrument, until his electric shocks became less and less and finally disappeared. Thus the nerve cells in the brain governing the electric organ were completely tired out and could no longer work. Without giving these nerve cells time to recuperate, or to gain new energy by assimilating food from the blood vessels, the animal was killed and the cells compared under the microscope with those of the second torpedo which remained completely at rest. Thus we had side by side under the microscope, the overworked fatigued cells, and those in a perfectly normal resting condition, which had a full supply of energy. The problem was to determine not so much any outward changes in the form and shape of the cell, as its interior mechanism. Definite changes were found between the two sets of cells, changes that throw some light upon the all-important problem of how the nerve cell does its work, and carries on its life operations.

It should not be understood, however, that the fallacious view is entertained that comparative histology of the nervous system, any more than any other purely morphological study, can investigate function by merely studying shape and form. Such study is not adapted to investigate the *activities* of life. The phenomena of life are caused by mutations of energy. The analysis of life phenomena on the basis of energy should form the guiding principles of morphological studies. Morphology can get no deductive sweep over its provinces without a study of the cause of life phenomena—cycles of liberation and restitution of energy. Comparative anatomy of the nervous system must then be inspired by comparative or general physiology. Since the phenomena of consciousness may enter into the subject psychology also comes into play.

As a basis for future investigations of this department,

biological material has been collected quite extensively, more particularly marine forms.

Collections of material like these are not to be worked through blindly and merely to store facts. The facts sought for should be of qualitative rather than of quantitive value. The facts sought should be those that may be used, and to use the facts one must have some notion of the cause and effects in life phenomena. In short, comparative morphology should derive its guiding principles from the standpoint of general physiology. Morphology then becomes a philosophic study, involving the verification of causes and a fitting in of its facts with the *modus operandi* of life phenomena. Physiology contains the philosophy of morphology. Deeply impressed with this idea, I trust that comparative anatomy of the nervous system, in the plan of a coalition of sciences in psychiatric research, may be continually stimulated by the ideas of general physiology by carrying on some of its researches in the *marine biological laboratories*, such, for instance, as the one establised at Wood's Holl. During the summer season the department should transfer its work to such a centre and study the nervous system in closer relation to the general biological sciences. This branch of investigation is under the guidance of C. Judson Herrick, A. B., (Dennison University).

Chapter VIII.

DEPARTMENT OF CELLULAR BIOLOGY.

Cellular biology, lying rather remote in its field of study from the province of the asylum, those who are in touch with the insane may not wholly realize that this science forms one of the corner-stones in a rational system of investigating insanity.

The science of the cell has accomplished marvels within the past few years, and from the days of Schleiden, Schwann, Purkinje, Von Mohl and Müller vast strides have been made. Inasmuch as the whole body is a vast commonwealth of these tiny cells, some working together in a community, as in the kidney, other communities in the liver, and still others in the brain, it ought to be easy to understand that the whole ultimate solution of the workings of the body, both in health and disease, resolves itself into a study not only of the *statics* of the changes but of the *dynamics* of the individual cells themselves. Yet as Loeb, who has a profound insight into the true philosphophy of the general dynamics of life, points out* general physiology cannot be restricted to the study of special organs, nor to that of particular cells, amoebas and the like, nor can it be made identical with a study of cellular physiology unless we understand by the latter an inductive and deductive application of its laws to the *whole realm of life* phenomena. Virchow, fifty years ago, forecast that the ultimate study of disease processes, particularly in their beginning and essences, must be devoted to the cells themselves. The student of cellular biology looks upon the cell as a microcosm in itself, and his investigations have been so searching as to point to the path toward the solution of the problem of the physical basis of heredity. If the study of the cell would be rather of dynamics than that of statics, the path itself would be nearer in sight.

In studying the egg cell, just after it has started on its growth, to produce a new member of the species, the biologist has found that equivalent and equal amounts of

*Einige Bemerkungen ueber den Begriff, die geschichte und Literatur der allegemeinen Physiologie. Physiological Archives, Hull Physiological Laboratory, Vol. II.

a certain element of the cell are derived from both the father and mother. He has shown, furthermore, that these two equal and equivalent paternal and maternal elements are woven together, and by a most intricate process, distributed in equivalent amounts to every cell in the whole body. It is on this ground that Huxley says the entire organism may be compared to a web of which the warp is derived from the female, and the woof from the male. It is certainly wonderful to stand at last face to face with some intelligent and fact-supporting basis of the mechanism of heredity.

We can now have some glimpse of how immutable are the laws of heredity. This material—the germ plasm—transmitted in equal amounts from both parents to the new individual, will surely pass on damages incurred by the ancestors. If a man exposes his germ plasm to the poisonous influences of alcohol, or still worse, syphilis, such damage is not confined to his individual life only but passes on to the next generation. This damage plays a part in subtracting from the full development of the organism, especially in the most complicated tissue of the body, the nervous system. This subject of heredity is of great importance in the study of insanity, but it were well that discussions of heredity in insanity might more generally rest upon the scientific basis of our present knowledge of the germ plasm and the theories of inheritance. For if the theories be applied deductively to the phenomena of inheritance in insanity two benefits result. The facts are rearranged and marshalled in order. This being done it is to be expected that the theory will be tried and fortified. Light will then be reflected upon the theory from an inductive standpoint.

Cellular biology has also another province which cannot

be disregarded and that is embryology, which in a certain sense is correlative with the study of pathological states and conditions. The most reliable method of gaining knowledge of the architecture and function of the nervous system is to watch its growth in the successive stages of development of the embryo. Here we are able to realize the functional value of different parts of the nervous system, by studying their various stages of growth as the embryo passes through its phases of development. First, the lowest and most fundamental parts of the nervous system appear, which have to do with the mere organic and vegetative functions of the body. Little by little the higher and more complex parts appear in their turn, so that we can trace, in the growth of the embryo, chapter by chapter, the whole story of evolution in a recapitulated form. The particular value of this method lies in the fact that we are enabled to determine, in a general way, the function of different parts of the nervous system, as they make their appearance in serial order in the embryo; the lower and fundamental parts always come first, the highest and most specialized in function last. The early stages of this study of the embryology of the nervous system, naturally fall within the province of cellular biology, for it is in the developing egg that this science has gained its most brilliant achievements.

The province of cellular biology in regard to touching on the province of insanity, is so intimately linked with the scope of pathological anatomy that it is difficult to dissociate the two sciences, and discuss them separately. Briefly stated, *pathological anatomy*, or the science which treats of the structural concomitants of disease processes, *can make further progress only on condition of using the science of the cell.* I mean by the science of the cell not only a study of its statics but also of its *dynamics*. Cellular statics is only a stepping-stone to the elaboration of the laws of energy applied to the phenomena of life.

The department of cellular biology in the modern centres for scientific investigation of the insane is absolutely indispensable. The whole study of changes wrought by disease processes in the nervous system is absolutely dependent upon the principles and methods of cellular biology. Such a department is constantly consulted by the pathologist, and it is due to this department that he is able to interpret the changed condition of the brain in disease, which he views under the microscope.

Perhaps the strongest argument for the value of cytology or cellular biology in the study of the pathology of mental diseases can be realized when we perceive that Nissl's method itself is really an outgrowth and an application of the principles and exact methods of cellular biology to the nervous system. Without in the least detracting from the fame of its discoverer and the value of his great work, Nissl's method is to be considered more as an extension of the general cytological methods of cell study to the nervous system than as an innovation in a particularized technical method. If the application of Nissl's and similar methods to the nervous system be regarded in this light—as extensions of the methods of cellular biology and requiring a knowledge of the functional organization of the nervous system when these methods are used—they can be used broadly and intelligently in the investigation of the pathology of mental diseases, and are destined to accomplish startling advances within the next decade.

Nissl's method and its congeners should be viewed as methods of cytopathology which expose the morphology of the whole interior organization of the nerve cell in contradistinction to the crude and restrictive methods of the older pathological anatomy. These latter methods merely brought to light the external form and shape of the cells and gave an account only of the coarser and grosser morbid changes which were so far advanced as to be destructive, inducing obtrusive changes in the *external form* and *contour* of the cells. Nissl's and the cytological methods generally (for Nissl's method of staining is but one of many of these cytological methods), exposing the *internal organization* of the cells, present a hitherto entirely hidden view of structural changes parallel to the whole *normal* and *pathological metabolism* of the nerve cell; that is, as far as the process can be comprehended from a morphological standpoint unaided by the conjoint application of the general physiology. It is herein that the Nissl type of method is so valuable for investigation of the diseases of the nervous system, for we are able to see the initial stages of disease process in the *interior* of the nerve cell. But to speak of seeing stages of disease process because through the microscope we see certain alterations of structure in cells is to fall into a somewhat prevalent error of accepting descriptions of abnormal structure for explanations of pathological life activities.

Disease is a process not an entity. One must have a dynamical and not an ontological conception of it. The phenomena of disease are expressions of cycles of liberation and restitution of energy. One must have something more than a knowledge of altered structure in cells to comprehend the real process of disease. One must have a conception of the true cause of disease, namely, energy and the play of factors which enter into its mutations which are food supply and external energy liberating impulses or stimuli, as they are called in the domain of life. The man who sticks to what he can observe through the microscope in diseased tissues will have a hard time attempting to see energy and its cycles of liberation and restitution which constitute disease processes. Therefore he hardly gets an inkling of what the whole great drama of disease really means. By the aid of the microscope the process can be indirectly verified but not directly observed. If he would know the meaning he must possess the key to the understanding of the dynamics of life, which is, that life phenomena (excepting consciousness) are mutations of energy. In short, he must use the genius of general physiology for the mental elaboration of his facts. For this science has for its province the deductive and inductive application of the laws of physics and chemistry to living matter. It should be clear, then, that we mean by cellular biology a more comprehensive standpoint than cell morphology. Its standpoint is morphology plus *general physiology*.

The whole life-history of all forms of mental and nervous disease, except the last chapters, goes hand in hand with morbid changes in the internal organization of the nerve cell. When the morbid process has gone on so far as to induce defects in the external configuration of the nerve cell, it marks the closing scenes of its life. The nerve cell then passes over into the grave; for these changes are beyond reparation; its life-history is closed, its cycles of metabolism have ceased; its delicate mechanism subservient to the expenditure and restitution of nervous energy is irrevocably damaged and no further expenditure of energy is possible, except that issuing from the organic dissolution of the cell manifested in non-nervous energy or energy liberated in the form of heat, or chemical reactions of organic destruction. One can realize how much, then, in the morphological basis of the life-history of mental and nervous diseases has been ignored in the study of late destructive lesions of the nerve cell by the crude methods of pathological anatomy, and how much is to be learned through the services of cellular biology in donating to psychiatry and neuro-pathology the Nissl type of methods of investigation.

Future advances in the whole province of the pathological anatomy of mental as well as nervous diseases depends upon the application of the principles and methods of cellular biology.

One exceedingly important topic also falls within the province of cellular biology, when linked with the investigation of medical sciences, and this is the study of disease processes artificially induced in the lower animals. The lower animals, even down among the invertebrates, offer opportunities for elucidating wider and more fundamental truths concerning the cell microcosm than the higher animals, especially man.

Experimental work on these lower animals made up of relatively small colonies of cells in a simpler and more elementary form, constitutes one of the most fruitful fields of inquiry as to the behavior of the cell in the environment of disease processes. In man, and even in the higher animals, when disease processes are experimentally induced, the conditions are much more complex, so much so as to hide frequently the fundamental changes of the reaction of the cell as an individual. Since man is simply an aggregation of cells, the same general laws that govern the individual cell must also govern his organization.

The experimental induction of disease processes in the lowly and more elementary organism with a view to study the reaction of the cell in abnormal environment of pathogenic stimuli, under the simplest conditions, seems again, at first glance, to be straying from our proper pathway, the study of insanity. This, however, is not so. The nervous system is made up of myriads and myriads of these same kind of cells, marvelously compounded into one organic whole. No other cell in the whole body can compare with the nerve cell for complexity of shape and internal organization. It is not sensible to attack the problem of cell-dissolution by selecting for study the most complicated cell in the whole body. It is plain that the proper way is to study first the course of disease processes in the simpler cells. Having learned this, we can forecast what ought to happen in the complicated differentiation of the ordinary type of somatic cell into a nerve cell, and be prepared to understand what the changes in the nerve cell mean when it comes in contact with abnormal stimuli inducing disease processes.

As a general rule it is to be expected that the fundamental conceptions of cellular statics and dynamics are to be verified or induced by a study of the lower order of cellular units in the organization of the complex media of life, such as man, or in the whole scale of life itself. For the external complexities of stimuli are simpler and more controllable in the study of the lower orders of cellular units. The neuron furnishes a striking exception to the generally safe rule in solving many problems in ascending from a lower to a higher order of complexities. The neuron is the highest differention of the cell complex, yet its study furnishes an insight in the energy basis of the phenomena of life incomparably more valuable than any other order of cells in the whole organism, or, indeed, in the whole range of life organisms. In the course of evolution it proved most useful to the organism to have in the neuron the maximum of dynamics. In seeking for the laws of the transmutations of energy as the *modus operandi* of life phenomena the study of the bacterium, the amoeba, the unicellular organisms and lower metazoa is indeed valuable, but still I think that no member of the cellular hierarchies ontogenetic or phylogenetic sheds such a flood of light on the cycles of energy liberation and restitution unfolding life phenomena, as the neuron. The study of the dynamics of the neuron furnishes the key to the energy theory of life. We may see, therefore, that a study of the highest units in life may unfold generalizing principles whose grandeur and sweep are but dimly outlined in the study of a lower order of units. The phenomena of life are most emphasized in the activities of the neuron.

We may be sure of one thing, that the nerve cell was at one time much like any of the simpler cells of the body, and that all these complex structures in the nerve cells are not new creations or *fiats* in its evolution from the simple cell, but are merely devices and modifications of the structures present in its simply organized ancestor. In other words, a cell of simple structure like the general type of somatic cell, in undergoing the phylogenetic evolution into the nerve cell, has not created new and specific elements, in order to accomplish the duties of a nerve cell, but has used its old and elementary structure and by differentiations and modifications made them fit to accomplish the offices of the nerve cell. In studying the cytopathology of the nerve cell one should hold in mind that, notwithstanding the marvelous adaptations of the cyto-reticulum and cyto-lymph of the nerve cell wrought by evolution out of these fundamental cytologic structures common to all cells, the nerve cell should not be considered apart from the other cells of the body. The neuron is not a specific creation, it is after all a cell; its structures are homologous with other cells of humbler organization in the body, and obeys the same general basic laws governing normal and pathological metabolism like its humbler associates in the cellular body colony.

The laws which govern pathological processes (and some day these, it is to be hoped, may be expressed in terms of cell energy) operate uniformly for all of the cells of the body. The laws make no special reservations or exceptions for the cells of the nervous system, even its most highly organized spheres. Disease is one general process, but as this process manifests itself in a great variety of phases corresponding to a Protean expression of symptoms often grouping themselves in a distinct type as a distinct malady, one, therefore, must be careful not to wrongly consider the phases of the single process as individual entities and distinct processes. Various kinds of inflammations and cellular degenerations and other pathological processes should not be spoken of as individualized processes, they are merely phases of the same general process.

The more cellular biology, including both cellular statics and dynamics, is used in the study of pathological anatomy, the less tenable becomes the idea of individualizing specific morbid processes with specific diseases. When, therefore, we are attempting to study the changes in the brain, we must never forget to summon to our aid cellular biology to help us understand the meaning of the pathological processes in the nerve cells.

Let us glance for a moment at the reciprocal benefits to be gleaned from a broad union of the medical and biological sciences and especially at the *influence of the marine biological laboratories on the progress of medicine.* The value of the application of the theories of evolution as guiding principles in pathology and patho-anatomical research as well as the light reflected back on the theory of evolution urgently demands a strong, well studied rendering. I can only call attention to the subject and cannot in the least fulfill the task.

It might seem, at first sight, as if psychiatric research were straying far away from its legitimate territory in extending its work into the marine biological laboratory, but it is a sad mistake to draw lines between the medical and the biological group of sciences. Psychiatric research stands in need of the study of the neuron in its cellular individuality, and such study should be judged by general knowledge of the cell theories.

Under Professor Whitman's inspiration the Marine Biological Laboratory at Wood's Holl, Mass., is fulfilling the ideal of correlating the biological sciences. It is a school where, happily, a spirit of philosophy is in the foreground with guiding principles for the gathering of facts.

The Marine Laboratory of the United States Fish Commission, at Wood's Holl, opened again for scientific work through the broad-minded spirit of the present Commissioner, Mr. Bowers, is seeking the same ideal under the direction of Professor Bumpus, an ideal which we hope will not be abandoned, but striven after with even greater perseverance.

If the ideals of these laboratories were carried a few steps higher, by including pathology in the family of biological sciences, the plan would be still more perfect. The phenomena of pathology and the facts of pathological anatomy are in great need of guiding principles from the theories of inheritance; of variations; of cellular adaptations: and, above all, from general physiology. For these phenomena and facts are still in confusion and have not found their full value from the standpoint of the energy basis of life phenomena. In pathology and pathological anatomy facts are greatly in excess of ideas wherewith to estimate their value.

The great question behind the study of structure is what animates the mechanism, and how is it animated, in normal or abnormal life? The question is not answered by reducing the structures to smaller and smaller units of divisibility. In passing from the grosser topographical investigation of morphological changes in organs to the individual cell or changes in the particles of the cell, pathological anatomy only evades the question. To face the problem of the *modus operandi* of disease process, one must approach the phenomena of disease from a more general standpoint and reflect on the fact that the degenerative changes in a cell are things left behind after something else has departed. *The thing which has disappeared is energy.* The changes in the dead cell do not constitute the process of disease any more than the charred remains of the gun powder constitute the explosion.

To face the problem of the dynamics of life, and this is the ultimate problem of vital phenomena, one must conceive that *all phenomena of vitality are modes of motion and that in life the same laws are operative as in the inorganic world.* In the problem of the activities of life the process of storing latent energy in the cells by assimilation and the liberation of energy by the overcoming of resistance by other impacts of energy or stimuli must be taken into consideration. These processes cannot be grasped by study of structure alone. Other methods of investigation than the purely morphological, and different trains of thought, are required.

Yet I do not want to undervalue the study of morphology in disease. It is of the greatest value, if inspired by philosophy and a proper general groundwork for inference from the general principles of energy as the basis of life phenomena. I merely emphasize *the importance of studying function and structure hand in hand.* Medical sciences will receive their impetus from the biological sciences, from the standpoint of *function, of energy manifestations.* General physiology is indeed the central inspiration of the medical and biological sciences.

One must make use of deduction and formulate the problems before working at the facts. If the idea is wrong, its imperfections will be brought to light in the process of verification by the facts. It is better to use the facts in pathological anatomy to test theories than to have an expectation of finding some truth by delving out facts at random.

Physiology as it is generally taught in medical schools has also much to gain from the suggestive touch of the marine biological laboratory, for this form of physiology is special in its character, it is addicted to the investigation of the function of particular organs. Its specialization is somewhat at the expense of the comprehensive sweep of *general* physiology, which is not limited to organ, tissue, amoeba cell or individuals, but works out the laws of the dynamics of living matter throughout the whole realm of life.

At the same time it is to be hoped that the marine biological centres will turn their attention and devote more of their time and work not only to dead, but also, if not principally, to living cells. It is somewhat strange that studies of the living cells have been so much neglected by the morphologist, or that he had not more extensively observed the living side by side with the dead cells, and varied the environment of the former with regard to restitution and liberation of energy. It is unfortunate that many are content to believe that descriptions of mechanism are explanations of its activities.

The advantage, however, of joining the medical and biological scientific communities in a more intimate philosophical relationship by no means confers a one-sided benefit on the medical group. The biological federation of sciences and the student of evolution miss a great opportunity in neglecting comparative pathology, human pathology and pathological anatomy.

In disease the expenditure of cell energy proceeds at a faster rate, and the restitution through assimilation at a slower rate, than in normal cell life. The process is not essentially different in normal and pathological states. The difference is only in degree. In pathological processes, greater degrees of resistance are overcome, deeper levels of energy are unfolded and more intense stimuli come into play. Into the flux of all these factors enters the play of change, both of kind and degree, of the cellular food supply, and also the factor of predisposition diminishing the resistance present in normal life. The play of all of these factors opens a sweeping vista into the structural and dynamical life-history of the cell which is but dimly outlined to biologists who restrict themselves to the observation of the normal cell.

In disease external circumstances act on the cell, change the environment and call forth corresponding adaptation in the cell. In this experiment we find an opportunity of studying cellular adaptations and variations that throw some light on the theories of evolution. One point of reciprocal benefit to pathology and biology in the marine biological laboratory is an interweaving of the theories of evolution with pathological phenomena. The pathologist can hardly expect any ultimate explanation of pathological processes without having a general knowledge of the theories of evolution and heredity combined with the broad working hypothesis of the mutations of energy, applied to pathological and patho-anatomical processes.

On the other hand, the student of biology may have a flood of light reflected upon the theory of evolution by including the domain of disease within his horizon. The theory of evolution takes account mainly of external configuration or gross morphology with respect to phylogeny. Variation and its growth with selection must have similar underlying modifications in the cells. The fundamental factors creating phylogenetic variations in cells are food supply, the storing of energy in the cell and energy liberating impulses or stimuli, which overcome resistances and set free the latent energy in the cell. The play of all these factors in creating variations in the cell is most prominently brought to the surface in the observation of pathological cellular processes. The principles of evolution should be carried more extensively into the province of the cell considered as a chemical machine, through which energy is stored from food supply and liberated by the agencies of stimuli overcoming resistance.

The germ plasm is to be considered the same way. Changes in environment is the great modifying factor in evolution. These disturb the external circumstances, modify both food supply and stimulus, and hence modify the cell itself, and determine the persistence of the variation as an adaptation. Since the phenomena are mutations of energy, morphology alone cannot fully grasp them. The great field for future studies in evolution is pathology, or rather pathological physiology.

The study of evolution has passed to the investigation of the cell. Much of this, although greatly centered about the egg cell and its immediate progeny in ontogeny, also takes account of phylogeny. Still the study of the cell is not sufficiently illumined by the energy basis of life phenomena. The study of evolution depends too much on morphology, and too little on general physiology.

At present there is a growing demand for a sounder and more extensive inductive basis for the study of evolution. This is realized for instance in the work of DeVarigny. In the problems of life, however, too great a reliance on the inductive method is unsafe, because of the mutiplicity and conflicting nature of the proximate causes. The causes themselves have to be regarded deductively. In extending the study of evolution into the domain of pathology there is opportunity for a keen, powerful weapon of thought in an intimate union of both methods. On the one hand is the ultimate cause, energy, the guiding principle for deduction; on the other are the most magnificent experiments of nature in disease processes, as a basis for the inductive method. By the reaction of each method on the other, I think that the expectation is not exaggerated that evolution would gain a new standpoint of thought as startling as that of Darwin's.

There is a particular reason why the study of evolution should consider human pathology, because of our knowledge of man's psycho-physiological life. Pathology (the study of the dynamics of disease process) and pathological anatomy (the study of the structural alterations in disease) are in much the same position as the biological sciences at the time of Darwin. If a second Darwin could arise for the pathological sciences, he would find the storehouses of these sciences almost bursting with facts requiring generalization. The Darwin of pathology will find the suitable environment for his genius in general physiology. From its principles, he will descend upon the phenomena of pathology, and the facts of pathological anatomy, and weave out of them not only a classified, but a consistent body of knowledge in relation to the laws of energy. He will not be confused by founding his deductive basis on the proximate causes of disease, the energy liberating stimuli, but will have the ultimate cause of morbid processes—cell energy—as a commanding eminence to survey the majestic drama of disease. The uttermost details of structural changes will not be of vital concern to him, nor will the finding of the uttermost explanation of the source of energy itself interfere with the consummation of his ordained work. He will conceive that the laws of evolution pertaining to the organism as a whole also hold sway over the individual cells. He will perceive that the same struggle for food supply in the outside world goes on in the body in the growth of its units. He will see the perishing of the weak cells in disease and the survival of the stronger ones with greater degrees of resistance to liberating impulses. In brief, this man will possess a two-edged weapon with the deductive principle of energy on one side, and the great experiments of disease as an inductive standpoint on the other. With it he will wrest out great victories for pathology and perhaps still greater triumphs for the theory of evolution.

If the pathological anatomist would borrow a suggestion from the theory of evolution with its fundamental principle of the struggle of organisms for food supply, he would get a broad hint of the explanation of hyperplasia. He would at least see the hollowness of certain glib phrases which simply gloss over the difficulties.

The physician, the clinician, the practitioner whom the "scientific" laboratory pathologist regards as unscientific stands nearer the fountainhead of disease and is in a far better position to observe and follow the energy mutations of pathological processes than his colleague, the pathological anatomist. This which seems at first sight rather strange, if not paradoxical, is not at all surprising. For the reflective physician is really a physiologist, or to make a rather unnecessary distinction, a pathological physiologist. He observes the living phenomena, and manifestations of liberation of energy are obtrusively and dramatically put before him every day in rise of temperature, convulsions, œdema, delirium, the epileptic fit, and manifold other phenomena of liberations and restitutions of energy, called symptoms. He has an idea, vague and unformulated though, of the coming to the surface of the energies of life in disease. The pathological anatomist, however, sees nothing but the husk and the shell of something that has gone. He sees hieroglyphics graven on tissue or cell, but he is not able to interpret them until he knows of the invisible force that wrote them.

I think, then, that the influence of a closer union of biology and evolution on the progress of medical sciences becomes deeper and more important the further we go beneath the surface of things, the more we realize that the great inspiration to scientific progress is in new ideas, new trains of thought, and altogether in the subordination of observation and experimentation to guiding principles.

If the general subject of pathology profits by affiliation with the ideas governing biological research, psychopathology must gain as well, and likewise the subdivision of pathology which is concerned with nervous diseases. The marine biological centres at Wood's Holl concentrate a wide diversity of attention on the biological sciences. Representative men in all provinces of biology from nearly all the prominent universities in the United States gather at these centres. By means of lectures, conferences, seminars, individual discussions, ideas are exchanged and the results of research compared. The danger of isolation in work is warded off. Fortunately as this Institute is but a few hours away from these centres, and as they are essentially summer schools, no practical difficulties stand in the way of profiting by the far-reaching influence of the biological sciences upon the progress of the medical sciences and especially on psychiatry. We have recommended, therefore, that during the summer season the departments of cellular biology and comparative histology of the nervous system should transfer their work to these biological centres of research.

A most unfortunate gap lies between cellular biology and the pathological anatomy of the human body—cytopathology—a term but newly coined. I do not hesitate to say that the overlapping of cellular biology and pathological anatomy opens the richest of all domains for the future progress of medical science. If our endeavors to bridge over these two fields of science, so that they may work hand in hand, be made plain, I need say little more to defend the importance of cellular biology as one of the most powerful factors that contribute to successful organization of a centre for scientific investigation of the insane.

The department is under the guidance of Arnold Graf,* Ph. D. (Zürich).

CHAPTER IX.

PATHOLOGICAL ANATOMY, BACTERIOLOGY AND PHYSIOLOGICAL CHEMISTRY.

The departments of Pathological Anatomy, Bacteriology and Physiological Chemistry are so intimately linked together in the investigation of insanity that they may be dealt with collectively.

Pathology being the science concerning the origin, course and results of disease, had very simple beginnings. At first evil humors were supposed to gain access to the blood and to cause the departures from health. If we translate the term "humors" into the modern expression of toxic substances circulating in the blood, the older pathologists are not so far from the truth as regards the proximate causes of disease. But whence the humors arose and how they gained access

* As these sheets are passing through the press we are struck by the sad tidings of Dr. Graf's untimely death. This is a deep loss to the science of biology, especially in the field of cytology and cytopathology. Dr. Graf's great work, "Hirudinien Studien," including his theory of the physiology of excretion is being published by the Leopold Carolina Academy. His last work, Studies on the Nucleolus, will be edited by Professor T. H. Montgomery, and appear shortly. His work on fatigue of motor neurons in certain chelonians, his researches in the cytology of the human nervous system in a case of a criminal executed by electricity and his studies on the subject of the excretion of metaplasm granules in the neuron under pathological conditions, the latter undertaken conjointly with another investigator, are left unfinished. Unfortunately these latter works are left as fragments, and it may be impossible to collect them for record. An account of Dr. Graf's life and genius is now in preparation.

to the blood was all guesswork and speculation, and "humoral" pathology was a mere makeshift to define an unknown something which circulated in the blood and set free the phenomena of disease. In later days those who were concerned in the investigation of disease processes observed with the naked eye what they could of the changes in the body after death from any given disease, and were able to see that many of the symptoms corresponded to gross, coarse and destructive changes in the various organs. As the microscope improved, and ideas of the cell as the elementary unit of the whole body became more definite and coherent, the pathologist studied these coarser and grosser changes in the organs under the microscope, but even here he saw results rather than beginnings of the processes. The observation of some final members of a series of *morphological* changes could hardly give any idea of the whole complicated range of the antecedent members, much less furnish any explanation of the true cause of these effects and its *modus operandi* in manifesting abnormal *function* in disease. Professor Prudden quotes a line from Oliver Wendell Holmes, in which the work of the earlier pathologist is compared to an inspection of the fireworks on the morning after the show.

In those days the practising physician was also the pathological anatomist. He combined both functions. He observed disease in the living and sought to find its havoc amid the body structures after death. His methods, however, were limited to the study of the topography of the lesions of the disease, and *not to the pathological processes themselves constituting it.* In short, he saw results, but knew not whence and how they came. For the origin of these morphological concomitants of disease processes can be found, not in the gross and terminal changes in great communities and masses of cells, but within the subtle recesses of the cells as individuals.

For many years the pathologist went along bewildered by the phenomena of inflammation. He was able to describe with much precision facts and observations, but he failed to understand their significance. Meanwhile cellular biology progressed with rapid strides and disclosed the marvels of the cell microcosm. The older pathological anatomist was in somewhat of a Rip Van Winkle attitude pending this march of cellular biology, and awoke in bewilderment at finding that all his work in the study of morbid structural changes stopped short of the real origin within the cell as an individual. He neglected the beginning and saw only the end.

The advances in cellular biology are destined to give an enormous impetus to the future investigations of pathology. What, perhaps, puzzled the pathologist the most, before he had learned to peer into the cell microcosm for the solution of his problems, was the great number of important and serious diseases of everyday occurrence which seemed to leave no traces whatsoever upon the body. This was especially the case in many diseases of the nervous system. It was exceedingly perplexing, for instance, to understand how such a dramatic and dreaded attack of the nervous system as hydrophobia should leave no traces after death. The same might be said of epilepsy and many forms of insanity. These the pathological anatomist set down as diseases "*sine materia*" or cast them into the makeshift category of "functional" or idiopathic diseases. To-day, however, we are in a more fortunate position to understand why it seemed that no traces were left in the body from such serious diseases as these. The *secret lies in changes in the very inmost recesses of the nerve cells themselves.*

The older patho-anatomist concerned himself but little with the cell as an individual. If its shape, form and contour were unchanged, it passed muster as sound and normal, without regard to a whole world of changes which might be present in its internal organization. In scrutinizing the effects of disease he looked at the outside of the cell, and not at its vital organization within, as one might attempt to understand the contents of a book by looking at its binding. Thus, naturally enough, the knowledge of the structural changes of a whole host of diseases, particularly of the nervous system, was passed over unnoticed.

It is different to-day. The pathologist has borrowed the searching methods of the modern cellular biologist, who looks into the inner constitution of the cell and beholds a world of changes in the cell in general, and in the nerve cell in particular—changes which until now were entirely ignored. At the present time the anatomist in stuyding the diseases of the nervous system is actually peering into the mechanism of life operations going on in the laboratory of the cell. He is endeavoring to study the changes in the body of the nerve cell—changes going hand in hand with its assimilation of food and elaboration of energy. He is able to study the changes which happen within the cell when its food supply is interrupted or interfered with. Through this refined study of the organization of the neuron cell body—the headquarters of operations in the cycles of neuron metabolism—we realize that the oft recurring phenomenon of nerve fibre death so characteristic of subacute and chronic diseases of the brain and nervous system, is not the result of primary processes in the nerve fibre itself or in the surrounding neuroglia elements, but is entirely the secondary effect of lesions in the interior of the cell body.

When the food supply of the nerve cell is by slight increments qualitatively or quantitatively diminished, or, on the other hand, the nerve cell expends more energy—in states of pathological fatigue—than can be recruited from the food supply in the blood plasma, the nerve casts off *dead material* which is removed by the lymphatics. The excretion of these particles—*the metaplasm granules**—is most important in presenting a physical basis and a measure of the slow destructive pathological metabolism of the nerve cell which is such a prominent factor in the genesis of very many mental and nervous diseases. When the nerve cell begins to excrete these particles it is an indication of a lack of balance between the crude food supply of the cell from the blood vessels and the expenditure of energy. This *excretion of the nerve cell* is also the indication of senile degeneration, and it is most interesting to view this indication of senility of the nerve cell advancing prematurely in a host of mental and nervous diseases where the expenditure of energy of the nerve cell has been of a pathological and persistent character.

The excretion of the mataplasm granules is an indication of the slow, gradual and long continued liberation of neuron energy. The appearance of these granules seems a sure indication that the descending metabolism has gained vantage over the ascending process and little by little lower and lower levels of neuron energy are drawn off. Hand in hand with this the neuraxon dies. First the peripheral end dies and ascending metabolism becoming

* Van Gieson: Toxic Basis of Neural Diseases. State Hospitals Bulletin, 1897. To be continued in these ARCHIVES.

continually of shorter range the death of the fibre from lack of food supply from the neuron cell body continually approaches the cell body. In the decrease of the range of restitution of energy a shorter length of the neuraxon can be supplied with energy. In peripheral neuritis, in tabes, in general paresis, in amyotrophic lateral sclerosis, in pernicious anæmia, in chronic alcoholism and under many other conditions numerous observations of the excretion of metaplasm granules from the neuron cell body confirm my conception of the nature of nerve fibre death.

The excretion of metaplasm granules from the neuron cell body means that the tide of neuron energy is slowly ebbing away. Each incoming wave of restitution of energy may indeed almost rise to the level of the preceding outgoing wave of liberation of energy, but in time, if there be no turning point where flood outmasters ebb, the neuron is marked for destruction.

The most important bearing of the discovery (unless by this time it be well known) of the excretion of the neuron under pathological conditions is the indication of deficient food supply. This is a factor of profound importance in the genesis of mental and nervous diseases, and is also of extensive application. During life we have at present no adequate means of determining the factor of deficient food supply to the neuron cell body, nor can we fully realize how often mental and nervous diseases depend upon this factor which virtually means declining capacity or the storing of neuron energy. In the excretion of metaplasm granules from the neuron cell body (and especially in motor cells, *the migration of the nucleus*) we have a new and very delicate proof of deficient food supply for the nerve cells. If in the future we shall be able to determine a means of indicating the excretion of the ganglion cell during life by the tests of the physiological chemist,* another discovery of the utmost practical importance will be added to this great question of the variations of food supply for the neurons.

I do not hesitate to say, therefore, that the *metaplasm excretion* of the neuron, the working out of its significance and that of the *migration of the nucleus* are discoveries not only of considerable theoretical, but also of practical importance. Of course the length of the fibre and the relative amount of work done by various neuron aggregates enter into the discussion of deficient food supply of the neuron. These points, although of much importance, can here only be hinted at and must be taken up elsewhere.

The pathologist is now busily seeking the degenerations occurring in the interior of the ganglion cell when exposed to poisons, especially to those generated in the great mass of general body diseases. In the poisoning of the nervous system from general body disease, the pathologist is able to show changes within the interior of the nerve cell which go hand in hand with the liberation of neuron energy in the delirium in typhoid fever, influenza, sunstroke, etc.

We are able in these days, thanks to the aid of cellular biology and its methods, to study the changes in the nerve cell wrought by fatigue, to watch the nerve cell grow old and perceive the signs that indicate the approach of its decadence. It is particularly interesting to watch the *premature senility* and shortening of the life of the nerve cell by chronic *alcoholism* and *syphilis*.

Definite laws of the fluctuations of neuron energy, the

* I have already suggested this problem to the Department of Physiological Chemistry and the work is under way, beginning, if possible, with the chemical identification of the neuron metaplasm.

expenditure of energy of the diseased nerve cell, the restitution of energy in recovery from disease, with their concomitant psychomotor manifestations formulated at this Institute are helping to clear away the mystery of the modus operandi of a whole host of mental and nervous diseases.*

The rise of bacteriology is too familiar and of too recent occurrence to need any detailed account of its relation to pathological researches in the nervous system. Bacteriology in its great public practical services to sanitation, its application by boards of health in the prevention of infectious diseases, the almost miraculous practical outcome of bacteriological studies in the anti-toxine treatment of diphtheria, its great service in protecting and forewarning the healthy against disease, all these one cannot help acknowledging as being of great benefit to humanity. The services of bacteriology show clearly that it is an important department in medicine for finding the proximate causes of morbid processes and thus indicating practical measures to the prevention of disease.

The department of bacteriology, it should be expressly understood, does not undertake to carry on researches in the whole domain of the biology of bacteria in general, but restricts its energies to useful ends in the study of insanity, namely, the identification of bacterial poisons associated with nervous or mental diseases. This department, however, keeps in constant touch with the broader aspect of bacteriology in general, as a science, and keeps cultures of many forms of bacteria for the purpose of determining, experimentally, the action of their poisons upon the nervous system of animals.

* Vide "Neuron Energy and its Psychomotor Manifestations," ARCHIVES, Vol. I, No. 1. A further study will appear in the ARCHIVES in monograph form.

When the pathologist beheld the action of these disease-producing bacteria, he at last began to approach the proximate explanation of many morbid processes. He now sees that these disease processes are liberations and restitutions of static cell energy initiated by chemical reactions between the cell molecules storing latent cell energy on the one hand and forms of energy liberating impulses embodied in poisons and other pathologenic stimuli. The cell stores latent energy by assimilation in building up its complex molecules. This energy is set free by impacts of kinetic energy acting on the cells from without. These external impacts of energy acting on the latent cell energy are stimuli or energy liberating forces. These stimuli are comparable to the spark which ignites gunpowder and liberates its energy. The spark is not the true cause of the explosion. The true cause is the latent energy of the gunpowder itself. The spark is a liberating impact. It is an impingement of active energy on latent energy overcoming its resistance and thereby setting it free. If the latent energy of a cell is easily liberated the resistance is correspondingly small. If the cell energy is liberated with difficulty, that is, if it requires a strong liberating impulse or stimulus, its resistance is great. Bacterial and other poisons overcome resistances of latent cell energy beyond the range necessary for response to the stimuli of normal physiological life. Bacterial and other pathogenic poisons are energy liberating impulses. They seem to operate on the cell by chemical reactions whereby the cell molecules are reduced to lower and lower orders of complexity of organization. With each descent in the tearing down of the cell molecules more energy is liberated and also more resistance interposed. Predisposition, which means a diminution of resistance, is a pivotal factor in pathological ranges of energy liberation, but the consideration of this factor is full of difficulties. *The process of disease should in the future be discussed in terms of fluctuations of cell energy.*

As a rule bacteria are not harmful by their mere mechanical presence, but on account of the powerful poisons which they give rise to. It now seems that inflammation is the expression of a conflict between the cells of the body on the one hand and the bacteria with their associated poisons on the other. The idea of a conflict, however, in inflammation between cells and bacteria is somewhat unfortunate, for it hides a broader explanation of the phenomenon which can be better understood by thinking of the relation of cells to their food supply—and the energy basis of disease processes in general.

The conservative nature of disease processes is most beautifully shown in inflammation. Inflammation is found to be a protective mechanism in the struggle of the organism for its life existence, and is the outcome of a long series of adaptations on the part of the cell. This protective mechanism against the proximate causes of diseases extends throughout the whole scale of animal life, even to the amoeba. Were it not for this protective adaptation on the part of the body cells, the highly organized forms of animal life, as well as the human race, could not exist, for by long odds the conditions producing disease are in the ascendant over those contributing to normal life.

We must not, however, overestimate the direct bearing of bacteriology on the study of insanity. Bacteria are very seldom directly responsible for mental maladies, and comparatively rarely for nervous diseases. They do not attack the brain directly, nor is it to be supposed that there are specific bacteria for individual diseases of the nervous system. The action of bacteria in damaging the nervous system is indirect. The brain is so well protected against their incursions, that they generally attack some other part of the body. The nervous system is injured by the *poisons* which bacteria give rise to. The bacterial products enter the circulation or lymph spaces, come in contact with the nerve cells, and poison them, that is liberate neuron energy. Not an inconsiderable share of diseases of the nervous system in general take their primary origin in bodily diseases. These general body diseases, such as typhoid fever, pneumonia, syphilis, small-pox, influenza, scarlet fever, etc., either by their poisons or by interference with the food supply of the nerve cell, cause it to degenerate. In short, bacteriology and pathological anatomy are closely interrelated. It is not alone sufficient for the pathologist to recount the subtle changes occurring within the nerve cell in disease and render an opinion, to the effect that these changes are due to the action of a poison. We must know what the poison is, and where it comes from. In the solution of this question, bacteriology and physiological chemistry are indispensable.

The physiological chemist goes far deeper than the bacteriologist in identifying the proximate pathogenic stimuli. The devotees of medical science, particularly of pathological anatomy and pathology, are turning in eager anticipation to the science of physiological chemistry for a deeper solution of the question of concomitance of chemical changes and cell degenerations. What the pathologist observes under the microscope even in the most delicate changes of cell organization, is really far short of a causal explanation of disease processes. Behind all these morphological changes in the cell is a series of most complex chemical adjustments, and behind these adjustments or concomitant with them are the cycles of liberation and restitution of cell energy.

All diseases as well as normal processes run parallel to cycles of chemical analysis and synthesis in the cell. Cell chemistry is still in its infancy. Its great motive is to furnish the chemical steps of normal and pathological metabolism of the cell concurrent with the corresponding cycles of energy. It is by means of this science that we can have any hopes of discovering the chemical composition of the cell; the reactions of the cells to poisons; the nature of these pathogenic poisons themselves, their origin, their interference with the food supply provided by the blood to the cells for the elaboration of their energy. When all these problems are solved, the abnormal changes in cells, seen under the microscope, will be more fully explained, because we shall be better able to assign to such changes their dynamical valuation. The province of physiological chemistry is the connecting link between the concomitance of pathological cycles of cell energy liberation and restitution on the one hand and structural changes on the other. Beside each increment or decrement in cell energy I imagine a corresponding chemical (or physical) change, and beside each chemical change, a corresponding physical alteration. But what we see of structural changes under the microscope must be very fragmentary counterparts of the chemical changes parallel to the energy fluctuations in the cell.

As physiological chemistry advances it would seem that a more complete series of the chemical concomitants of cell energy fluctuations would be furnished than can ever be given of the structural effects of these fluctuations of cell energy by morphology. While physiological chemistry is striving to fill up the gap between structural changes and cell energy fluctuations, it seems best to apply the theory of cell energy deductively to pathological cell changes and describe these changes as effects of cell energy fluctuations.

Physiological chemistry has its specific *rôle* in the investigation of insanity. Few of us realize the fact that at every moment of our lives poisons are generated in the body itself, poisons which in health are taken care of and eliminated. When, however, some slight hitch occurs in the delicate equilibrium of the chemical reactions going on in the complicated laboratory of the body, widespread havoc may occur. A poison generated within the body may escape into the blood, and while it may do comparatively little damage to the more lowly organized and more resistent body cells, it may still harm the sensitive and highly organized nerve cells. Of all parts of the body the nervous system is the most sensitive to toxic substances. The sensitivity of the nervous system to pathogenic stimuli make it a delicate index of the presence of poisons generated within the body itself.

The conviction is daily gaining ground that many forms of insanity which arise so insidiously are initiated by self-poisoning. The microscope may show us traces of these poisons on the cell, but their source and nature can only be discovered by the methods of physiological chemistry. The microscope is, no doubt, powerful, but it cannot penetrate into the depths which physiological chemistry can reveal. Beyond a certain region of morphological research into the mechanism of the nervous system, the microscope alone proves an utter failure. These poisons generated by the body are of such subtle origin that it would seem almost beyond the power of science to identify or trace them. The physiological chemist attempts to identify them by examining the secretions, or the blood. If unable to identify and separate them directly from other components of the body fluids, he is still able to indicate their presence—he injects the body fluids into animals and watches the physiological effects by which he is enabled to tell whether the body is generating poisonous matters.

In identifying the poisons associated with bacteria the researches of the physiological chemist have been attended in many instances with brilliant success. In tetanus, for instance, the bacteriologist at first identified the bacteria of tetanus, has studied their whole life-history and habits, and has even found this germ in the wilds of Africa, where the natives smear their arrows with mud of certain swamps which become partially dry during the summer season. This earth contains the spores of the tetanus bacillus, and thus the strange fact explains why the victims struck by their arrows often die of tetanus.

The physiological chemist, however, has gone further than this. He has succeeded in isolating the poisonous principles associated with the tetanus bacillus, and is actually able to separate them in the form of a powder so that one might carry round in his vest pocket a real liberating agent of tetanus, were it not so sinister a substance and so extraordinary a poison, for 0.065 of a gramme is absolutely fatal to animal life. Such a poison transcends in intensity almost anything that we know of among drugs and inorganic poisons. A little of the tetanus bacillus poison goes a good way, and it is not unlikely that many other bacterial poisons are almost as powerful. The poisons formed within the body itself seem to be less fulgerant in their action; they are mild in intensity and operate insidiously; but, unfortunately, they offset this mildness by their tendency to remain persistent. This presents a great barrier to the restitution of the nerve cell, for it is deprived of an opportunity to rest and recover its pathological expenditure of energy.

Seeing that not an inconsiderable proportion of mental diseases is initiated by the action of poisons upon the nervous system, especially those of general bodily disease, it is of the utmost importance to trace them and use, as far as possible, practical measures against them. I think, therefore, that pathological anatomy, bacteriology and especially physiological chemistry need no further words of explanation of their place in the investigation of insanity.

We must not, however, fall into the error of believing that the researches of pathological anatomy, bacteriology and physiological chemistry, no matter how brilliant or searching they are, can give any explanation of insanity. If proximate causes of certain phases of insanity, mere neuron energy liberating impulses, are discovered in the form of toxines and bacteria, the *modus operandi* of abnormal mental life is not all explained. The discovery of these proximate causes is, no doubt, of great benefit from the standpoint of treatment, but this, however, is far from being sufficient, something more remains to be accomplished. We must *explain* the phenomena as well as the agents which set them in operation. Least of all can the microscopic study of fragmentary morphological traces of the ebb and flow of neuron energy furnish so much as an inkling of abnormal mental life. It is really time that the idea of patterning psychiatric research after medical investigation were abandoned.

If we wish to gain an explanation of insanity it must be plain that the first and main thing to do is to study insanity itself, to investigate the living phenomena of abnormal mental life. This the branches of medical research cannot accomplish. The phenomena of consciousness are beyond the grasp of medical sciences, and it is a delusion for medicine to pretend that it can investigate mental life. This belongs to psychology. Psychological investigation of abnormal mental phenomena themselves will furnish guiding principle of the *modus operandi* of insanity. Once this is accomplished the various medical and biological branches immediately fall in line; their investigation subserve a purpose and can be guided to bear on the explanation of insanity. Psychiatry can go on indefinitely under the guidance of the medical conception of research and profit only by piling up inco-ordinated details of anatomical, physiological and chemico-physiological observations, if this be of any real scientific profit, and still be no nearer to any great co-ordinating principle of the phenomena of abnormal mental life. The most that can be gained by the present medical methods is the discovery of some of the proximate causes without attaining at any real insight into the nature of the psychopathological processes that give rise to the symptoms of mental diseases.

With all of these wonderful avenues of investigation recently opened in the research of nervous and mental diseases, when it comes to the *explanation* of the phenomena of abnormal mental life, neither the pathologist, nor the physiological chemist, nor the bacteriologist can go beyond the mere description of facts and observations. *The real meaning of the great majority of all the changes in the nervous system, in mental maladies, the significance of the manifestations associated with these changes during the life of the patient can only be made clear through the science of psychopathology.*

The futility of attempting to understand the workings of consciousness by the medical conception of becoming familiar with its mere utensils,—through the study of anatomy, physiology and chemistry is charmingly expressed by Professor Ewald Hering's fine essay "On Memory and the Specific Energies of the Nervous System:" "The nervous system, and above all, the brain, is the grand tool-house of consciousness. Each one of the cerebral elements is a particular tool. Consciousness may be likened to a workingman whose tools gradually become so numerous, so various, and so specialized that he has for every detail of his work a tool which is especially adapted to perform just this kind of work most easily and accurately. If he loses a tool he still possesses a thousand other tools to do the same work, although with more difficulty and loss of time. Should he lose these thousand also he might still retain hundreds with which he can possibly do his work still, but the difficulty increases. He must have lost a very large number of his tools if certain actions become absolutely impossible."

"The knowledge of the tools alone does not suffice to ascertain what work is performed by the tools. The anatomist, therefore, will never understand the labyrinth of cerebral cells and fibres, and the physiologist will never comprehend the thousand-fold action of its irritations, unless they succeed in resolving the phenomena of consciousness into these elements in order to obtain from the kind and strength, from the progression and connection of our perceptions, sensations and conceptions, a clear idea about the kind and progression of the material processes in the brain. Without this clue the brain will always be a closed book."

"We can, indeed, compare the brain to a book. A

book is anatomically a number of rectangular white leaves, bound on one side, and marked on their pages with numerous black spots of different form and size. Under a microscope the leaves will be seen to consist of delicate fibres, and the black spots of minute black granules. A chemical analysis will show that the leaves are cellulose and the spots carbon and resinous oil. If all has been investigated and ascertained with the utmost accuracy, we do not know, in the least, why the black spots are arranged just in this and in no other way, why some spots are large and others small, why some occur frequently, others rarely, why the single leaves follow one another in this and in no other order, and altogether what the book really *means*."

"Whoever wishes to know what the book signifies must know what is the function of the specific energy of each single letter and of the individual energy of each single word—in short, he must know how to read."

The interpretation of the book is indeed sealed to purely medical methods, notwithstanding the amount of analysis that may be performed by the mainstays of medical research. To know how to read the book we must turn to the science of the phenomena of consciousness—psychology—and above all to the science of the phenomena of abnormal mental life—psychopathology. The medical sciences can never furnish the key to the book. Once psychology and psychopathology yield the key, the medical sciences have great value, the analysis of the form of the letters, the ink, the paper, yield a meaning and have a purpose.

A curious division has arisen between the practical fields of nervous diseases and mental diseases, a split that has created a very unfortunate and artificial gap in scientific research. However important it may be from a practical standpoint to separate nervous diseases, that do not interfere seriously with the intelligence from mental diseases that require a radically different treatment, the division in the scientific investigation of the two sets of diseases has been a distinct drawback in the progress of knowledge of each. The progress of knowledge of mental maladies has suffered the most in being considered a field of investigation apart from that of the nervous diseases. The damage in nervous diseases involves the lower and more simply constructed parts of the nervous system, and were the understanding of these simpler conditions applied to the domain of mental diseases, greater advances would have resulted. One distinct aim of the Institute in many of its departments is *to bridge over this artificial hiatus in scientific study between nervous and mental diseases.*

Now we find that the nervous system (even in its highest spheres) behaves like other parts of the body in the presence of disease processes. It was suggested in the preceding section, that the nerve cell may exercise a protective agency against hurtful stimuli by retracting its arms, which also provided a period of rest for the cell to recuperate pathological expenditures of energy from its food supply. When the hurtful stimulus becomes more intense, as in the case of poisons coming in contact with the nerve cell, notwithstanding the higher organization of the neuron, it behaves just like its humbler associates in the liver, kidney and elsewhere. It may undergo changes in its internal organization in contact with the poisons of disease; its food supply may also be interfered with. We then perceive, under the microscope, signs of degeneration of the nerve cell as witnessed in other parts of the body, when their cells are exposed to the influence of poisons.

But even under the influence of poisons, the nerve cell has a wonderful degree of vitality and a large capacity for restitution, when the disease-inducing poisons are withdrawn.

It is a very important view to consider that the brain behaves like other parts of the body in disease processes. Guided by this view we can avoid the pitfalls of error into which those investigators are apt to stumble, who are prone to think that the brain has its own disease processes radically different from those of the body in general. In studying the changes in diseases of the nervous system one must always hold fast to one fundamental truth, that the brain in disease must not be regarded as something apart from the rest of the body, and must not be isolated as an organ *sui generis* having inaccessible mechanisms and mysterious powers.

Whether in health or disease the nerve cells are like other cells only more highly organized. They must obey the laws of cell life in general. For it must always be borne in mind that even the highest constellations of the brain are not composed of elements distinct from the humblest parts of the nervous system, not even different from the simplest nerve that pursues its pathway anywhere in the body. The fundamental structure of the constituent elements is the same everywhere whether in a simple nerve trunk or in the noblest and highest regions of the brain itself.

Enough has been said, perhaps, to indicate the very comprehensive character of pathological research at the present day, and the fact has been emphasized that patho-anatomical process in the nervous system, and above all the brain should always be considered in the light of analogy of the general patho-anatomical occurring through the body at large.

The study of patho-anatomical processes in the nervous system then, in this Institute, must always be guided by a most comprehensive knowledge of these same processes occurring throughout the whole body. It is, however, extremely difficult for any one individual to have a working knowledge of the morphology of disease processes in the body in general, and at the same time know enough of the nervous system to extend into this field the broad conceptions of *general* pathological research.

The application of pathological anatomy to psychiatric research is liable to be shorn of its full value. The opinion seems to be held that a single individual can command the whole sweep of pathology in centres for psychiatric research. The idea still hangs on that patho-anatomical research in psychiatry is to be given over to the specialized pathological anatomy of the nervous system. As a matter of fact the whole field of pathological anatomy is needed. In centres of psychiatric research then, it is best to provide for a co-ordination of the several fields of pathological anatomy by two or three workers in this branch who can pursue the several subdivided special lines of investigation and yet correlate them in order not to lose track of the generalized influences of pathological anatomy as a whole.

Taking our own institution* as an example, we may say that the department of pathological anatomy is somewhat at a disadvantage in not having a sufficient working force to cover the whole field. We have, practically, but one associate to take charge of the manifold bearings of this branch of the investigation of mental and nervous diseases and of its interrelation with other departments in the Institute. Another representative is needed in

* For details of the status of working force in Department of Pathology and division of labor in this field, see original report.

this field of study, especially in collaborating and extending the work among the members of the staffs of the hospitals, for most of our colleagues in the hospital *choose pathological anatomy as their favorite work.*

This insufficiency of working force in the department of pathology, has also been a very serious drawback in the acquisition of that particularly valuable kind of material for investigation which is not to be found within the asylum. The opportunity for acquiring this material, so valuable in the investigation of insanity, largely determined the seat of the Institute in the great metropolitan city of the State. This material is derived from autopsies on cases in which the nervous system is damaged by the great host of general bodily illnesses. The making of autopsies; the acquisition of autopsy material of nervous diseases; the preservation of this material with the requisite great care and detail, all involve an enormous amount of work, and we have been unable to take full advantage of the very opportunity, which led to the inauguration of the Pathological Institute in New York city, namely, the acquisition of material and facilities for the study of the first stages of insanity, the importance of which was emphasized in the introductory paragraphs of this paper.

Finally, let us be quite clear as to the distinction between pathological anatomy and pathology, a distinction which, unfortunately, is too often lost sight of. Pathological anatomy is concerned with the study of the structural changes associated with disease process. Pathology is the study of the disease process itself. Cell changes or other structural lesions are effects, traces of the process of disease. Pathology has for its province the study of the phenomena, the manifestations of the abnormal function in disease. Pathology is a study of the *dynamics* of disease, whereas pathological anatomy is an investigation of its *statics*. In studying disease we should not be content to stop with making observations of pathological structure. This is but a small part of the problem. We should endeavor to go beyond this and explain the facts from a consideration of abnormal function. Pathology is the guide of pathological anatomy. Pathology, however, to be a trustworthy mentor of morbid anatomy, should be inspired by general physiology, the science of the general laws of the physics of function.

The comparison of the work of the earlier morbid anatomist to the inspection of the fireworks the morning after the show is still quite true to-day. The patho-anatomist of the present day is not far from the same position. In the contrast of the great progress of his deeper powers of analysis with the crude methods of his predecessor, the pathological anatomist of the present time is, I think, too prone to think that the force of Holmes' epigram has lapsed. In connection with the enormous amount of work rather heedlessly running into the channel of morbid structural changes it is quite as forcible as ever, and it will remain so as long as the study of morbid structure piles up its facts in delirious haste with too little reflection that only through the study of abnormal function can these observations have any broad interpretation. I mean by the study of abnormal function, not only the abnormal function of particular organs, but also the general principles of function in terms of cell energy, the province of *general physiology*. Pathological anatomy should turn to pathology, and this latter science to general physiology for the intrepretation of the structural changes in disease.

The same old problem, as to the cause and *modus*

operandi of the lesions, is still before the patho-anatomist of the present day. He has approached a little nearer to its solution, that is all. Like his predecessor, he still comes around after the show is over. The only difference between the two is that at present the inspection of what is left of the fireworks is much more extensive and penetrating. The patho-anatomist has passed from the observation of topographical lesions in organs and tissues to the minutiæ of cytological changes. Even so, the display is over. The living phenomena are gone and with them the key of explaining the meaning of the structural changes. This consists in expressing the structural changes in terms of function, of dynamics. Only the results, side products, impresses of the active phenomena of abnormal function are witnessed under the microscope. The observation of the finest minutiæ in cell structure is a long way off from the explanation of the energy process accompanying or rather giving rise to the cytolytic lesions.

Since the brilliant discoveries of bacteria and their toxines, and with the progress of seeking autogenous substances, the patho-anatomist of the day may be lead more than ever to think that the application of Holmes' epigram is a thing of the past. The difficulties of explaining the nature of pathological metabolism lie before us not behind us. The bacteriologist and the physiological chemist share honors in pointing out their discoveries as the causes of disease. The pathological anatomist points to the changes in cell, or organ, or tissue, when these causes are introduced into the body. It would appear, then, that the work of all three explained the *modus operandi* of the phenomena of disease. From the labors of the bacteriologist and physiological chemist, it would seem as if we had on the one hand the causes, and the other hand, in the observations of the anatomist, the effects. The causes, however, are not the true essential cause; they are only proximate causes; and the effects are only a part of the operation of the true cause. The things which the bacteriologist and physiological chemist have found, although discoveries of brilliant importance in practical utility, are merely what touches off the fireworks; what sets free the pyrotechnic display. These bacteria and toxines, while greatly advancing our knowledge of the nature of disease, are merely sparks, as it were, which ignite the fireworks. Hence, these three scientists are rather prone to fall in with the idea that each particular disease corresponds to a particular set of fireworks, which can only be ignited by a particular kind of a spark. This is an extremely shortsighted view of the problem. A knowledge of the igniting impulse or a study of the remains of the fireworks or both combined, do not explain the process of combustion.

Because his two co-workers have discovered the agencies which set the fireworks free, the patho-anatomist must not lose sight of the fact that he is still inspecting the fireworks after the show is over. *The man who actually witnesses the display is the physician, the clinician*, but even he, on reflection, will confess that his methods are not searching and that he perceives only a small part of the process and its manifestations. In fact what is needed is the wand of the science of general physiology to guide pathological anatomy, bacteriology and physiological chemistry. *The great science of life in disease and health is general physiology, the science of function.* There is no need of qualifying physiology in its application to the study of abnormal function. For function in general is the central province of general physiology. The duty of this science is to formulate function in terms of energy. When general physiology enters more extensively into the study of disease we shall see that the process of disease is one of mutations of cell energy and realize more fully the deep meaning which is conveyed by Sach's substitute in the term *energid* for the rather meaningless word—cell.

The department of Pathological Anatomy is under the charge of Henderson B. Deady, M. D. (Columbia University), and Bronislaw Onuf, M. D. (University of Zürich).

The department of Bacteriology is under the guidance of Henry Harlow Brooks, M. D. (University of Michigan).

The department of Physiological Chemistry is guided by Phœbus Levene, M. D. (Imperial University, St. Petersburg), and S. Bookman, Ph. D. (University of Berlin).

Chapter X.

PATHOLOGICAL PHYSIOLOGY.

I have endeavored to show in some of the preceding sections that in these days of great specialization and subdivisions of the fields of pathological research, it is out of the question for any individual to have the capacity to cover the entire territory. Twenty, perhaps even ten years ago, when methods of investigation in pathological research were in a comparatively elementary stage of development and were used uniformly for the investigation of disease processes in all parts of the body, a single individual mastered the whole territory and was a general practitioner and pathologist to boot. He could observe symptoms during the patient's life, bridge over the chasm of death, as it were, and write the sequel of the story of the disease by observing the changes in the organs under the microscope. At the present time, the problems of pathological research have grown vastly more complex The examination of different constituents of the body forms distinct and specialized territories of research, each having particular and intricate methods adapted for its special purpose, which cannot be used uniformly for the investigation of all parts of the body. Thus the changes in the blood alone, associated with disease, constitute a distinct field of research with specialized methods of investigation, and within the past few years an extensive literature has grown up emphasizing the importance of specialized micro-chemical investigation of the blood.

The study of the general changes linked with disease processes throughout the body at large, including the study of tumors, constitutes a very wide field of research, and is more or less subdivided into distinct branches of investigation. The study of morbid processes in the nervous system constitutes another field of pathological research, which is in turn subdivided into many specialized branches of investigation. The investigator who would explore this field must first traverse the domain of general pathological anatomy, must then learn the intricate architecture, construction and function of the nervous system, in order to apply to it his knowledge of the general nature of disease processes.

Pathological physiology in its turn constitutes a highly important and specialized domain of pathological investigation. Studies in this field of research that seek to investigate pathological function on a basis of physiology and induce disease processes experimentally require special skill in conducting operations on animals, and of watching the abnormal physiological manifestations of the animal after the experiment has been performed. It can be seen then that this territory merges over into that of physiology. If pathology be restricted to the mere observation of *changes in form* within the organs and their constituent cells during the processes of disease, its power of investigation terminates quite abruptly in very many directions; in fact it almost loses its whole dignity and philosophy as a science. Most pathological laboratories are not laboratories of pathology, but of pathological anatomy. We must not only observe the alterations in form and structure within the cells during disease processes, but also interpret structural changes by the study of the changes in the *functions* of the organs and of the cells themselves. In brief, pathological physiology takes into account the *abnormal physiology* of organs and cells when exposed to environment simulating that of disease. This most important branch of research in pathology, respecting the abnormal physiology of the organism during disease, is best conducted from the standpoint of general physiology, and should make constant use of the methods of experimental pathology. Pathological physiology fills up the gaps in the knowledge of disease processes gained by studying them in the human subject alone. These gaps are indeed wide and deep.

Anatomy deals with the structure of the normal organism. Physiology is the science of function.

Each of these two great sciences of life is specialized on various provinces, which need not be considered here except as relating to the divisions made in the study of disease. Both of these sciences become subdivided into specialized fields of inquiry depending upon the normal or diseased condition of the organism. Thus we speak of normal anatomy and histology as the branches which investigate the structure of the normal organism. Similarly normal physiology is used to designate the study of normal function. Pathological anatomy and histology investigate the structural changes concomitant with the process of disease. Pathology is the study of function in disease, and is, therefore, really identical with physiology. Pathology is an application of general physiology to the investigation of changes of function in disease. Pathology, however, is so often confused with pathological anatomy that it seems well to emphasize the fact that the great and guiding study of disease is not one of structure, but of function. The investigation of the disease process is not pathological anatomy, it is a physiological study and has a higher dignity as a science than morbid anatomy. In fact pathology should be the guiding science for pathological anatomy. In order to bring into greater prominence the necessity of physiological methods of investigation into the province of the study of disease, we have, therefore, used the term pathological physiology—the physiology of disease. Throughout this chapter the application of pathological physiology has been given a rather specialized character in being limited to the study of abnormal functions of particular organs in disease, both in the human subject and by experimental work on animals. In the future, after this department becomes established and grows, we shall endeavor to have its work guided by the broad principles of comparative or general physiology—the study of function in general on the energy basis of life phenomena. We should remember that the process in disease is not different in nature from the processes of normal life. In disease normal physiological processes take on a wider range. Cycles of cell energy liberation and restitution in disease are not different from the cycles in normal life. The range of the oscillations of the cycles are merely wider.

If the normal physiologist would have a flood of light shed upon normal function of cells and organs he should study the process of disease. *It is only through a study of the abnormal, the pathological, that we can hope to understand the normal.* This fact is not sufficiently understood by the devotees of the various normal "*ologies.*"

As normal physiology deals with the functions of the different tissues or organs in the normal organism, pathological physiology investigates the abnormal functions in the diseased organism. But the questions which pathological physiology has to decide are much more complicated than in those of normal physiology, because of the protean aspects of disease and the great variety of phases of the pathological process. Disease is very seldom so simple a phenomenon as the expression of the abnormal functioning of a single organ of the body. The body is a united whole, and the various organs are so indissolubly interrelated that abnormality of functioning in one organ may produce a widespread effect on the functions of the other organs. Disease is a complex whole of abnormal functions of various organs, although primarily it may result from the departure of a single organ or tissue from its normal functions, chemistry, and structure. In disease the pathological physiologist is, as a rule, confronted with a whole complex group of abnormal functions of several organs, and he has to sort out and differentiate how far the abnormal functions of each organ contribute to the general symptomatology and to discuss the interrelation of the abnormal functions of the several organs.

Before long he should, from the general biological study of function, discuss the functions of diseased organs in terms of cell energy. This will give the key to the explanation of the morphological changes in disease.

We must not be carried away by the fairly widespread example of centering pretty much the whole of scientific inquiry of medicine about the microscope, the crucible and the culture tube. Let us keep in mind that clinical work, the study of the *living phenomena*, the strict scientific investigation of psychomotor manifestations, is just as much a great department of scientific research as those laboratory investigations in pathological anatomy, bacteriology and physiological chemistry. In fact, I think that the study of the living phenomena is far more important than the other studies, for the simple reason that only through the study of the living phenomena of disease can we arrive at broad, guiding principles to direct and interpret the work of the laboratory sciences. The study of the living phenomena then, far from being put in the background of medical science by laboratory workers should stand foremost; it forms the mentor and the guide of these other sciences.

Clinical investigations conducted on the strict basis of general physiology and psychopathology give a basis for deductive reasoning, for scientific co-ordination of the scattered facts of the laboratory sciences. The clinician, fortified by the great principles of general physiology, pathology and psychopathology, armed by the methods of scientific observation and experimentation stands close to the highest plane in medical science—the observation of living phenomena, the manifestations of disease. At present, however, the methods of the clinician fall short of this standard—they are not wholly adequate and searching. A whole host of phenomena slip out of his grasp or are but dimly perceived by him. Physiology, functional pathology and psychopathology possess the methods of studying the living phenomena accurately and comprehensively. By pathological physiology, functional pathology or simply pathology, I mean to indicate the study of life activity in disease by the methods of a science which considers such phenomena as manifestations of *energy*. Clinical research, based on the principles of pathological physiology, ought to take precedence over the other medical sciences, such as pathological anatomy, bacteriology and physiological chemistry, and to lead them in *thought*. The study of function in terms of energy *states the problems* which are to be verified by the statical sciences. Through the leadership of physiology dealing with the ultimate cause, energy, the scattered, disjointed facts of pathological anatomy, physiological chemistry and bacteriology will become scientifically useful and yield material that can be used for *theory*, *generalizations*, *laws*—the ultimate aim of scientific research.

Inasmuch as we are largely debarred from controlling diseased human beings for the application of physiological methods of inquiry, we must obviate these difficulties by inducing morbid function in animals. This will not invalidate at all the soundness of the *general principles* of the *modus operandi* of abnormal function. These general principles (the nature of excessive ranges of cycles of cell energy liberation and restitution, and the nature of stress or resistance of latent cell energy to stress removing impacts) we should determine first through comparative or general physiology. We shall then be in a better position to reason from these generalities respecting cell energy as to the nature of functions of cell communities in the particular organs and tissues. General physiology of disease comes first; special physiology of diseased organs should be pursued in the light of the former study.

Observation at the bedside is, to a large extent, a practical application of pathological physiology, but in most instances, such observation can only state the substance of the question as to the nature of disease processes, namely, the origin, cause and course of the disease, and is seldom able to answer it. Pathological anatomy may demonstrate that a given disease is followed by certain lesions in certain parts or organs of the individual, and may further show that the same lesions are always associated with the same disease, thereby making a certain relation between the two factors quite probable. But in order to change probability into certainty other methods of investigation are requisite. It is necessary to reproduce the disease experimentally and artificially in animals. If the pathological lesions found in a given disease can be initiated experimentally in an entirely healthy organism and disturbances in the functions of the organs similar to those of the disease result, the chain of evidence demonstrating the association of the symptoms and lesions is complete. This plan is one of the great aims of pathological physiology. Its highest motive is the interpretation of symptoms, abnormal function, in terms of cell energy. The greatest guide to the study of cell energy is the investigation of neuron energy. This is the key.

In this experimental method, not only in pathology but in all biological and natural sciences generally, lies the great power and advantage of modern methods of investigation over the old lines of research. In some instances, the experimental method in the study of disease may be applied to human beings, more particularly in methods of treatment. In fact, all of our present knowledge of the action of drugs has been gained through experiments in pathological physiology. In fever, for instance, the modifications induced in the abnormal functions of the body by antipyretics or a cold bath are useful applications of the experimental method in pathological physiology.

The opportunities for using experiment in abnormal physiological manifestations of human beings in disease are seldom afforded. Hence we have to make use of experiments on animals and compare the results with the phenomena of morbid processes in man. It may be said that pathological processes induced in animals cannot be compared with those occurring in human beings, for the organization of each is different. This is certainly true to some extent. There are, for instance, pathological processes of the gravest import to human beings, which, as yet, we have not succeeded in reproducing in animals, such as tumors, syphilis, epilepsy, the small-pox group, etc., and many diseases of the nervous system. There are again certain factors vaguely grouped under the terms predisposition and immunity which make an individual of the human species prone to a disease process and shield an animal from the same process, and *vice versa*. The idiosyncrasies of man to many diseases from which animals seem shielded go to show how much we still have to learn of predisposition, immunity, and the factors of heredity and vulnerability in disease. These facts in themselves, on the other hand, emphasize all the more the imperative necessity of the more extensive application of the experimental method in pathology, for the diseases which seem beyond the reach of the experimental method were formerly and are now precisely the very ones the explanation of which is most obscure and unsatisfactory. In many instances, fortunately, one is quite justified in considering the abnormal functions of the organ in an animal, when a given disease process is induced experimentally, as equivalent to the abnormal functions in a human being in that disease.

The cardinal functions of the corresponding organs are the same in all animals with higher organization, and the structure of these organs resemble each other very closely. If, then, having produced in an animal the same lesions corresponding to the ones found in the human subject, the animal is found to manifest the corresponding set of symptoms, the causal relations of the abnormal functions to the structural change rest upon a firm basis. This is the way that the brilliant and practical results of bacteriology have been achieved. Without the use of experimental pathology, bacteriology would indeed have been a sterile science in the practical domains of medicine. It would have resulted in a piling of Pelion on Ossa of mere facts of the life-history of bacteria, and their all-important pathogenic qualities would have remained comparatively unexplored.

We should not strive always to experiment on animals which, by the high and complicated development of their organization, are more or less related to human beings, but, on the contrary, greater extension of the experimental method in pathology should be made on the lower animals where the brilliant work of Metchnikoff has given the key to the explanation of the phenomena of inflammation. The less complicated the organization of the animal, the less complicated are its specific functions, and the easier it is to comprehend its structure and functions in either health or disease. But this field, experimental pathology in the lower animals, belongs to or is shared with the province of cellular biology and has already been alluded to. From these studies it will then not be difficult to progress to the understanding of the aspects of disease in more complicated organisms. For our purposes, experiments to produce disease processes on the more *highly organized animals*, belong more properly to the territory of pathological physiology. For the study of the specific functions of various organs a distinction between higher and lower realms of animal life is perhaps on practical grounds admissible; because the cellular biologist is more familiar with the lower forms of life than the special physiologist (medical physiology, physiology of man). From the standpoint of the general study of function, from the point of view of general physiology, such a distinction is wholly arbitrary and illogical.

When morbid processes are induced experimentally in animals, to find the equivalence of disease in the human subject, the services of physiological chemistry, bacteriology, and pathological anatomy, must be called upon; the secretions and excretions must be examined; the physical methods of examination used in the clinic or laboratory of normal physiology must also be taken into account. In addition, the tissues of the animal are to be examined by the microscope after death. To a casual observer, it might seem then that pathological physiology, having no methods of its own, could hardly be called an independent branch of medical science. This is as little true of pathological as of normal physiology. The aims of pathological physiology, the questions it has to study and decide upon are peculiar to this particular science, notwithstanding the fact that it works largely with methods of research used in other branches of medicine. Pathological physiology has a method of its own, namely, animal experimentation conducted along certain lines peculiar to this branch of science.

Like every other branch of medicine, experimental pathology or pathological physiology is closely, even organically, related with the other branches. It is a *connecting link* between *pathological anatomy*, *physiology*, *bacteriology* and *physiological chemistry* on the one hand, and *clinical medicine* and *hygiene* on the other. Its work is indispensable, not only for the progress in the treatment of disease, but also for advances in the highest art of medicine—the prevention of disease. Its greatest province is to guide the work of pathological anatomy, bacteriology and physiological chemistry, and furnish the standpoint for explanation of this work. Progress in modern surgery, in serum therapy, in the prevention of epidemics, in immunization, public hygiene and antisepsis owes a great debt to experimental pathology.

The study of the pathology of the nervous system is more dependent upon pathological physiology than that of any other system in the organism. All the other organs of the body differ from each other by anatomical structure and by function, while different parts of the central and peripheral nervous system have the same anatomical structure and still their functions are entirely different. We can hardly see, for instance, any morphological or chemical difference between some parts of the brain, the irritation of which produces contractions of the muscles; or other parts of the brain, the irritation of which produces contractions of the circulatory system, rise of temperature of the body, and so on.

The fact that every part of the brain has only to perform a certain part of work in the physiological division of labor in the nervous system, was shown first by Hitzig and Fritsch by the aid of animal experimentation. They irritated certain places in the convolutions of the brain with an electric current and always received contractions in certain muscles. These experiments having such a great theoretical importance for the understanding of physiology of the brain, played even a more important part in the pathology and in the localization of functions of different parts of the nervous system.

These experiments enabled the physicians to find in a living man a tumor of the brain, and the surgeon to direct the knife to its location with almost mathematical accuracy. Experiments of this kind corroborated the differentiation between focal and essential epilepsy, and it is to be hoped that the day is not far distant when the simulacrum of epilepsy may be artificially induced in animals through the labors of experimental pathology. If the simulacra of epileptic phenomena could be experimentally and permanently induced in animals, it would furnish the key to the explanation of this obscure process. All the facts which the pathological anatomist and physiological chemist have gained in the study of this dire malady give no explanation of the *process* that gives rise to the epileptic phenomena.

Animal experimentation has also proven that extirpation of certain portions of the cortical part of the brain always produces a degeneration in the same nervous fibres, proving thereby the neuron theory and showing the location and topographical distribution of different groups of functionally related neurons. Many more examples could be added, showing the value of pathological physiology for the study of the nervous system.

Far from being fit to investigate the phenomena of

consciousness, morphology and chemistry alone are not, and never will be, able to explain all the phases in the *function* of the nervous system, not only because we are unable to differentiate morphologically or chemically one pathological process in the brain cell from another, but also because the same pathological process of two different parts of the brain, if their functions are different, can have a different influence upon the organism as a whole. It is, therefore, not sufficient to study the morphological and chemical changes of the nervous system in its pathological state. We must also see what influence such a diseased nervous system has upon the different systems of the organism, such as the action of the heart, the blood pressure, the respiration, the general metabolism, and so on, as these all depend upon the nervous system, and must be changed when the latter is changed. Conversely the effects of changes in circulation, respiration, general metabolism and changes in organic and vegetative somatic functions upon the higher parts of the nervous system must also be taken into account. This latter topic must be studied by the pathological physiologist and psychopathologist conjointly.

We can illustrate our point best by the plan of studying the influence of drugs or poisons on the nervous system. Let us suppose that we introduce into an animal certain drugs that produce convulsions or sleep; no matter whether we find morphological or chemical changes in the nervous system or not, we will not know thoroughly the nature of the action of these drugs until we examine, by all the physical and physiological methods at our command, the influence of the drugs upon the nervous system itself and all other systems of the body, the action of which is regulated by and depends upon the nervous system.

From one particular standpoint, however, this branch of research deserves special emphasis, for it relates to some questions of ultimate and practical importance regarding the insane. One of the specific *rôles* of pathological physiology, in psychiatric and neurological research, lies in the *determination of the action of drugs upon the nervous system*, and above all the brain. It must be confessed, that in the treatment of the insane, our knowledge of the effects of drugs upon the metabolism of the nerve cells is very obscure. No one will deny that it is of the utmost importance to know what we are doing to the nerve cells in administering drugs to the insane. At present the knowledge of the action of the drugs given to the insane, is known simply by the general physiological effects, and not by the chemical reaction between the constituents of the nerve cell and the drug itself. Our knowledge of the action of drugs on the nervous system is empirical to the last degree. In epilepsy, for instance, I do not hesitate to say that in very many cases the administration of bromides on this entirely empirical basis, although relieving the symptoms, may actually in the course of time damage the nervous system severely. The bromides, if given continuously, may constitute an actual poison to the nerve cells, and in this disease one evil may be added to another, in that the ravages of the disease process of epilepsy is augmented by poisoning the nerve cells by a drug, whose action upon the delicate organization of the nerve cell is altogether unknown.

Epilepsy seems to be due to the action of some stimulus, which though mild in intensity, may, by its persistence, act in the higher spheres of the brain. This stimulus may come from a variety of places in the body. It may arise from the intestines in the form of a mild poison, which may escape into the blood from some departure in the complicated chemical operations attending digestion; it may travel up one of the many nerves of the body from some irritation which involves the ends of these nerves; it may be due to the irritation of a tiny splinter of bone pressing on the brain after a blow upon the head, etc. In an individual of inherent instability of the higher spheres of the brain, this constant stimulus finally causes a sudden dissociation of this part of the brain from the lower spheres beneath, by means of the retraction of the tentacles of the nerve cells. These nerve cells in the upper spheres of the brain become fatigued, through the constant reception of the stimulus, and retract their arms to avoid the noxious and offending impulse. But in the sudden retraction of the upper spheres of the brain, which grasp and control the lower portions, the energy of the latter is suddenly unbridled and loosened, and the epileptic fit results. Now it is quite probable that in deadening and benumbing these upper spheres of the brain by the use of bromides, so that they no longer exhibit a sense of fatigue to the stimulus much harm is being done. It is quite true, that the symptoms of epilepsy may be controlled in this way, but are we not poisoning the nervous system to gain this end? It were far better to ascertain the cause of the epileptic fit—the persistent stimulus coming from some distant place in the body—and attempt to remove this, rather than to injure still further the highest spheres of the brain, by benumbing with a poison their sense of fatigue.

If the large and continuous amounts of bromides be given to animals, as has been determined in some research work in one of the State hospitals, the result is the poisoning of the nerve cells manifested by the phenomena of degeneration. While the drug is not given in epilepsy in such poisonous amounts as in these animals, nevertheless it must act in the same way, though to a less degree. If a perfectly sane man were continuously dosed with bromides, it would seem almost certain that in the course of time he would begin to show a dissolution of the higher spheres of the brain, whose activities are concomitant with the manifestations of the highest forms of mental operations. It must appear, then, from this single example, how important it is to know the action upon the nerve cell of these drugs. Hence I would enter a plea for provisions in pathological physiology at this Institute, the more so as I have already mapped out an extensive series of experimental researches to determine the action on the nerve cell of the drugs used in the treatment of insanity.

In addition to the determination of this important and practical question by this department, many problems relating to self-poisoning in the body fall within its scope. Subtle disorders of a whole system of organs within the body whose duty is to maintain the blood in a proper equilibrium, may induce a poisoning of the nervous system with grave results. A very large share of our knowledge of diseases that spring from disorders of the organs producing the blood and maintaining its chemical and morphological equilibrium has been derived from the researches of pathological physiology. A large share of work still remains to be done in this field, and facilities for the experimental study of the relation of changes in these blood-producing organs, to poisoning of the nervous system in mental and nervous diseases, ought to be provided for at this Institute.

We have no one on the staff at present who has the requisite time or specialized training to undertake work in the field of pathological physiology. An associate in this department should be able, in addition to his own special investigations, to perform all the operations on animals desired by the other associates in the course of their researches, or to devise new operations and experiments as may be necessary in the course of psychopathological, pathological, bacteriological or chemico-physiological investigations. In addition to this, he should conduct all the physical and physiological parts of the examination, transfer and apportion the morphological, chemical and bacteriological material to their respective departments for detailed investigation after the experiment has terminated.

CHAPTER XI.

THE INVESTIGATION OF BLOOD IN INSANITY.

The investigation of the blood in insanity derives its importance as a distinct field of research, from the fact that this is the medium of conducting the food supply to the nerve cell. When the nerve cell works, it expends energy, and the elaboration of energy is carried on within the body of the nerve cells from crude food materials derived from the blood vessels. The theory has lately become more and more substantially founded upon facts and observations, that not an inconsiderable share of mental and nervous diseases are due to the actions of poisons upon the nerve cell. These poisons, which comprise a very large group, are sometimes bred within the interior of the body; they are often derived from bacteria and frequently taken into the body from extrinsic sources.

There is, however, great danger of carrying this explanation of the action of poisonous substances upon the nervous system, too far, and thereby underestimating the *equally important factors of deficient food supply and pathological fatigue of the nerve cell in the production of nervous and mental diseases.* In observing the actions of poisonous reagents upon the nerve cells, the concomitant impairment of *their food supply in relation to the work they perform* must also be jointly taken into account, particularly where the poisons, although mild in intensity, are of a dangerous character from their persistence and chronic action.

Investigations of the blood in the living patient, then, are of paramount importance, because *in changes in the blood we have a barometer, so to speak, of the fall or adulteration of the food supply of the nerve cells.* We have not only to consider the specific action of poisons upon the nerve cell, but the secondary factor of the interference and adulteration of food supply of the nerve cell which this poison causes by circulating in the blood. In one of the commonest forms of insanity—general paresis—constituting a considerable per cent of the patients in the hospitals near the large cities, the cause of the disease seems to be a slow, gradual, unrelenting process of diminution of the food supply brought by the blood, thus inducing starvation of the nerve cells.

The investigation of the blood in insanity has proved of such practical importance as to enable one to base on it therapeutic measures and to indicate the percentage of cases that may be benefited by a particular line of treatment. Herein is certainly a practical application of the value of investigation of the blood of the insane. If there be one factor more important than any other in the production of mental and nervous diseases, with the exception of toxic agents, it is the *quantitative* and *quali-*

*ficative impairment of the food supply carried in the blood vessels to the nerve cell.**

Much important work remains to be done in establishing more definitely the factor of impairment of food supply to the nerve cell in relation to the genesis of mental and nervous diseases, and the Pathological Institute of the New York State Hospitals can ill afford to neglect this branch of research, not having the aid of an associate in pathological physiology.

This once more may serve as a good example to show the inefficiency of the working force of the department of pathology, in having only one associate. Pathological research work covers so many specialized fields of inquiry that a staff of at least three associates is required. I think, however, that both pathological physiology and the investigation of the blood of the insane may be carried on by a single investigator.

To sum up, it is advisable, if not indispensable, that three sub-branches should be provided for pathological research in the investigation of the insane, each under the charge of a single associate. These sub-divisions are:

I. General pathological anatomy.

II. Special pathological anatomy of the nervous system.

III. Pathological physiology, including the pathological histology of the blood.

* Some of these details respecting the significance of the excretion of the metaplasm granules from the nerve cell in relation to deficient food supply and pathological expenditures of energy are worked out in my paper "The Toxic Basis of Neural Diseases," now in press for a future number of the ARCHIVES OF NEUROLOGY AND PSYCHOPATHOLOGY.

CHAPTER XII.

ANTHROPOLOGY.

The importance of heredity as a factor in the production of insanity has been hinted at several times in this text. In the previous section on cellular biology, attention was drawn to the fact that the advances in that science had set forth a working hypothesis for the physical basis of heredity; that the cell scientist had been able to select a certain element in the egg cell which in its fecundation was mingled with an equal amount of the same element from the sperm cell; that these two paternal and maternal contributions to the beginnings of the new being were intimately wrought together and distributed in equal amounts in the process of cell division to every individual cell in the whole organism of the new individual. Hence the new being bears the stamp of the characteristics of both parents.

The facts of the relation of heredity to insanity are to be interpreted only by applying to them the remarkable advances of cellular biology into the nature of the germ plasm and the investigation of variations in general through the study of evolution. The whole essence of the problem of heredity in insanity lies in a thorough appreciation of these researches of the germ plasm and of the nature of variations, and the psychiatrist who does not familiarize himself with these investigations in the community of biological sciences can hardly expect to gain any clear insight into the factor of heredity in insanity. The discussions of this subject frequently carried on with but vague and hazy recognition of the present status of cellular and other biological researches into the physical basis of heredity bears testimony to the isolation of psychiatry from all other branches of science. Psychiatry is its own worst enemy in not stepping forth and affiliating with the biological and medical group of sciences.

Changes in the germ plasm from either the paternal or maternal side or both, operate most powerfully to determine the weal or woe of the progeny, according to whether the nervous system grows up from normal germ plasm full, sound and stable, or contains as a result of pathological germ plasm some hidden, subtle, instability of the highest, most delicately organized and precious upper centres of the nervous system, endowed with the highest intellectual attainments and control over the brutal, credulous, immoral and aggressive sub-conscious self.

What are the agencies which damage the germ plasm and cause departures from its normal constitution? Precisely the same agencies, to a certain extent, which cause degenerations or induce disease processes in other cells of the body besides the germ cell. It is not a transmission of acquired characteristics. The germ cells are damaged principally by the same agencies as produce the variation and not necessarily or, only to a slight extent, the operation of the variations themselves. These agencies may be summed up under poisons and factors which depreciate the food supply of the body cells.

While in their whole life-history the germ cells are supposed to be set apart from the rest of the body cells for the distinct and sole office of continuously propagating the species, it is not possible for nature to colonize them so completely as to shield the germ cells from the damage inflicted by poisons or deficient food supply. Thus, for example, the poison of syphilis and the chronic and persistent poisoning of the body by alcohol, both of which seem to operate largely by diminishing quantitatively or qualitatively the food supply of the body cells, not only cause degeneration of the nerve cells, but damage the germ cell simultaneously and during the growth of the embryo inflict other ontogenetic variations also. This is the reason that the progeny of parents whose nervous systems are poisoned by alcohol and syphilis is notoriously defective in the weak organization of the superlative and most intellectually endowed spheres of the nervous system. For if a very slight defect or chemical change or a change in the configuration of atoms occur in the gigantically complex molecules, the germ plasm as a result of the action of these poisons, the effect in the next generaation will crop out in the highest and most complexly organized parts of the body rather than in the more lowly organized and comparatively undifferentiated parts. This is why the nervous system, and above all, its most lofty portions, are found wanting in perfection when the germ plasm is in a pathological condition.

According to the degree of pathological changes in the germ plasm do the defects of development of the progeny pass successively from higher to lower and lower planes of organization in the nervous system so that all grades of degeneracy and mental instability may be witnessed down to the weak-minded, the imbeciles, and idiots. The exceedingly complex molecular constitution of the germ plasm and the complicated process of reduction or halving of the germ plasm in maturation of the egg and sperm cells in relation to the action of toxic agents and deficient cellular nourishment is of such urgent importance that we ought to try to devise plans for the department of cellular biology to approach the problem from the experimental standpoint among invertebrates which afford good opportunity of applying toxic agents to the germ plasm.

During childhood such inherited incapacity of the energy of these higher parts of the nervous system does not always appear, unless the hereditary effects due to damage of the germ plasm or other ontogenetic variations be of a certain degree of intensity or persistence, for at this period such higher centres are comparatively little used. During adolescence and later life, however, when these higher centres of the nervous system are called upon for the greatest and most extensive expenditures of their nervous energy they may fail. We then perceive the outcropping of hereditary influences in a defective mechanism in the neuron to elaborate energy from its food supply. It becomes worse in the next generation, for the reason that this unstable brain energy in the first generation is liable to cause the individual to commit excesses; to set aside moral laws in decent, wholesome living, tamper with the nourishment of the body and introduce alcohol or other poisons into the circulation of the blood. Thus the germ cell in the second generation becomes still further degenerated in that it suffers from this exposure to poisons and imperfect food supply in the blood. Degeneration of the germ plasm in the second generation is liable to bring about pathological conditions in the nerve cells and other somatic cells disturbing the general metabolism of the body or inducing a craving for toxic substances (alcohol) in the third generation. This reacts upon the germ cells in the succeeding progeny and their degeneration is advanced in progressive generations. Degeneration of the germ plasm once established tends to set up a vicious circle increasing the degeneration in each successive progeny, unless somewhat mitigated by crossing with undamaged germ plasm. The third generation of such a succession is liable to become quite unstable in the energy of the higher portions of the brain which hold the lower spheres in check. It is from this or succeeding generations* that are recruited the inmates of the prison, of the lunatic asylum, of the reformatory and of the hospital for the epiletic and idiot.

We are, however, in such a backward state of general knowledge of all these phenomena among the masses that we cannot mitigate these agencies (better control of syphilis) or seize the earlier phases of generation psychopathies in the beginning, where they ought to be taken in hand, but must wait for the end, so that the State has to spend millions taking care of sickly and incurable degenerates. Spontaneous variation and environment must, of course, be taken into consideration in the march of degeneracy. But from whatever sources or combinations of these sources the degenerate and the candidate for the prison and the asylum springs, we must identify him and have knowledge of him in the earlier stages of his pathway.

Now as to the use and purpose of anthropology. The relations of anthropology to medical science are somewhat vague. No one seems to define clearly and exactly just what anthropology is to do, or what results we may expect from it; consequently one may avoid the ponderous definitions usually given and attempt to explain in simple language the use of anthropology in the science of medicine. Anthropology, in relation to the medical sciences, is simply a convenient term to indicate that two or three sciences are made use of collectively to study not

* Vide consideration of liberation of energy throughout successive generations in the paper on Neuron Energy.

only individual cases, but also large bodies of men. In this way the science simply makes use of anatomy, physiology and psychology, more or less simultaneously, in investigating normal and abnormal phenomena of human life.

Now our object with anthropology is to conduct these anatomical, physiological and psychological investigations, to determine the characteristics of men with abnormal nervous systems as compared with the normal. We wish to identify the degenerate; we wish to learn departures in the physical and psychical characteristics of men at various stages along the pathway toward the prison and the asylum. At the asylum we already know fairly well what departures the insane show from the average normal man. In the asylum, however, only the last stages of mental and physical abnormalities preponderate, and we depend on anthropology to work out the initial and intermediate stages in the course of degeneracy.

The first stages in the history of the degenerate, in a great majority of cases, is some defect of the germ plasm, and this or other ontogenetic variations give rise to the stigmata or marks of degeneration, both mental and physical, found in many of the inmates of the prison, of the reformatory, of the hospital for the epileptic and for the insane. In determination of the mental characteristics of degeneracy, anthropological investigation must be under the guidance of psychology and psychopathology.

Undoubtedly one of the most resourceful fields of anthropological research in its bearing on abnormal mental life is the study of the psychopathic and neuropathic criminal. The larger part of the sphere of what is called criminal anthropology really belongs to pathological psychology, since this possesses the methods of analyzing the abnormal mental phenomena shown in a certain proportion of criminals and can furnish the ideas, the philosophy of correlating the facts. The other side of the investigation in criminology, the determination of the physical abnormalties, belong properly to anthropology. A union of both lines of research would seek out both the psychomotor and physical departures in the criminal, their interrelation, and ultimately, laws and principles governing these variations.

By criminal anthropology we understand then a coalition of powers of research grasping at both the physical and psychical variations of the criminal in so far as his acts are symptoms of a defective organization or manifestations of pathological processes. Criminal anthropology, if I understand it aright, is the study of the *psychopathic* and *neuropathic** criminal. It is the study of those criminal classes only who are of a psychopathic or neuropathic nature.* This requires the combined work of psychology, psychopathology, anatomy and physiology. The sociological aspect concerns us very deeply in that it may furnish aid by contributing to some guiding principle of the research, but any specialized work along the lines of sociology lies outside of our sphere. Yet a co-ordinated study of the defective or diseased criminal ought to be productive of useful material for the sociologist to apply in his own especial problems.

It will be necessary from our standpoint to take a cursory glance at the development and aims of anthropological study (including above all the psychopathological investigation) of the diseased or defective criminal, for criminology has but comparatively few students. Students of this subject have a hard road to travel both as to the discouragingly difficult nature of the subject matter and

* See article "Neuron Energy."

the lack of encouragement and even the discredit they receive from other workers in science.

Possibly several things have combined to make criminal anthropology seem an unproductive or unattractive field of work. One reason for the lack of enthusiasm in the study of the criminal is that the science in itself is exceedingly young. It has barely had sufficient growth to establish ideals and plans of work. Consequently the study is somewhat vague in its outlines. It has not developed enough to map out pathways of investigation that others may follow with profit. Like many other branches of science dealing with life phenomena, general principles and working hypotheses are exceedingly difficult to ascertain by confining the research exclusively to the subject itself. It would be far better to study the pathological phenomena shown by some of the criminals where similar phenomena are greater in degree or are proceeding at a more obvious rate. One might then from such sources find some general theory, even if it be only provisional, to test the same in criminals and to see if the manifestations of the criminals are in accordance with the truths that have been learned about abnormal physical and mental variations elsewhere.

Another cause, perhaps, that has depressed the study is that among the laity especially, there is a feeling of distrust that the tendency of the advancing study of the criminal will be to ease him of responsibility and make crime attractive by making excuses for it under the guise of psychopathic maladies. In fact, the practical application of scientific analysis of criminal actions has often been abused in the halls of justice, and it is liable to be done often again in the future, as long as such evil systems of ascertaining scientific truths as that of "expert testimony"* prevail. Still in the long run progress in the study of criminology cannot fail to right such evils and to call for a less backward attitude of the law to regard the scientific side of criminal acts.

One other reason that may be given to account for the spirit of indifference in relation to the study of criminal anthropology is that its exponents have worked with fallacious methods of research.

The study of the criminal, in so far as he is neuropathic or psychopathic, hinges largely on the questions of the laws of human inheritance and human variations both physical and psychical; and these are the most vexed questions of the day. Progress has advanced so far only as to state them and point out the direction of the inquiry rather than to make an attempt to answer them. These questions point conclusively to the fact that the study of the criminal must be guided by general biological and psychological standpoints.

The obstacles in ascertaining the laws of mental and physical variations in man by focussing the study on the psychopathic or neuropathic criminal are altogether too great. In a study surrounded by fewer complexities, the method would be to assemble the principal external facts and by rising from them through the resources of the methods of induction arrive at the laws. But in criminal anthropology the difficulties are too great and transcend the powers of this method. It will be necessary to go to many outside fields of research in general biology and psychology to arrive at some standpoint for the guide of the investigation of the criminal.

To carry on work with the methods of induction experiment is necessary. In working with these methods we pro-

*See Van Gieson and Sidis "Expert Testimony," STATE HOSPITALS BULLETIN, 1897.

ceed by noting certain external phenomena or effects and by successively varying the surrounding circumstances, eliminate irrevalent pertubations until, finally, we arrive at the essential interrelation and correlation of the phenomena, that is, we discover their laws. Two conditions are requisite in this method, first to vary, by experimentation, the conditions surrounding the phenomena, and secondly to observe the particulars or analyze the components of the phenomena after the experiment. In the investigation of the criminal classes it is very difficult to do either. In the inductive sciences we can control the phenomena and hence are able to experiment. In the study of the psychopathic and neuropathic criminal classes it is rather difficult to employ the experimental methods. The student may note a whole multitude of facts, but to assemble them in orderly fashion, to estimate the relation they bear to each other, and to harmonize the relation of their segregate and aggregate value with our accredited knowledge and most certain experiences of other physical, mental phenomena will indeed be a hard task. The observer stands in danger of becoming lost and hedged in in his own mass of facts. From this standpoint the study of the diseased members of the criminal classes might go almost indefinitely and do little more than wander about in the maze of its facts without finding an outlet, for in the concentration of observation in the field of the criminal alone, no foothold can be promised for reflection and inference from the facts. Criminal anthropology no more than psychiatry or any other life science can be isolated from other fields of knowledge. Otherwise it loses its philosophy and its dignity as a science, and the finest and most patient of observation fails to be effective without the guidance of and reciprocal impetus to theory.

Perceiving then the present narrow standpoint of criminal anthropology, what other recourses are open? It is a question well worth while to inquire into; for the most important thing is to have some definite standpoint from which to conduct the lines of the research instead of catching hold of facts wherever we can or in whatever order they come along. One must endeavor to see through the relations of things instead of blindly hitting upon these relations through one successful effort in a series of chances. If a man is to make ten or twenty thousand measurements of criminals and the like, he is indeed expending energy and conducting close observations, but he also ought to have formulated clearly in his mind beforehand the precise object of these results and what use they are in relation to our stock of knowledge of mental and physical variations in man gained in other directions. If such a set of measurements are undertaken to verify a theory established by a substantial number of facts in human and general morphology, or from the standpoint of general study of the laws of variation and inheritance, no fault is to be found. But, on the other hand, if the investigator does the work at a venture and says that he cannot predict what startling results may not come forth from the computations, and has no well defined object in view except that he expects to hit upon some generalization from these bald columns of figures, I feel that it is not a high form of scientific work. It seems a little like the method that people use in solving mechanical wire puzzles by adjusting and turning them over in the hands until some one of the random attempts succeeds.

Criminal anthropology is as yet in too early a stage of development to seize upon the phenomena of its special field directly by the inductive method. It must first have theory, even if faulty, and make a little further progress on this basis in the marshalling of the facts. From this induction may be used then further deduction. By alternately passing from the one method to the other slow, gradual progress can be made. For this is the history of the first stage of growth of science in general. The facts lie before us all the time. But in the complexities surrounding the phenomena we are not able at first to unearth them and to have all at once perfected methods of inquiry to discover them. The most valuable facts lie beneath the surface and often defy the most ingenious methods of exploration. At the beginning, science has relatively few facts and these lie upon the surface and are obvious. Theories have to be invented and a *modus operandi* established for the succession of the phenomena from their antecedents and gradually the theories become more perfect.

To work out some guiding theories criminal anthropology needs the methods of deduction. In deduction we invent certain principles in the mind and descending upon the phenomena verify them to see if they agree with the hypothesis. In this way facts refractory to control and experiment, although yielding to observation, may be brought under the dominion of the hypothesis.

How can this deductive method be brought into play in criminal anthropology? We have two things to consider, the mental and the physical variations of psychopathic and neuropathic elements of the criminal classes, and we are to get at some principles for the co-ordination and succession of these phenomena. For the verification of the former set or phenomena, it seems best to select some opportunity where the psychopathies are more outspoken and not complicated with legal considerations, where the process is proceeding at a faster rate. In other words, it will be best to select the material with great care.

In some particular phase of the psychopathic process corresponding to definite sets of psychomotor manifestations, the components, although difficult enough to analyze, are far simpler for investigation than the actions of the psychopathic or neuropathic criminal, complicated as they are by sociological and legal considerations. We should study, therefore, some very carefully selected case furnishing the simplest and most controllable components in the process, as, for instance, from the group of neurasthenias, hysterias, amnesias, etc., or other forms of dissociations of consciousness. Working at such a case from the standpoint of a coalition of several branches of research on an inductive deductive basis, we may form some certain conclusions as to the *modus operandi* of the whole psychopathic process. These conclusions, increasing in value and truthfulness in proportion as we increase the extent of the study of the examples of psychopathic disease from which they are drawn, may be then used deductively to verify the phenomena of the defective or diseased criminal by specialized investigation. Such a scheme has at least some merit, for it proceeds according to method. It has a groundwork for construction and does not array the external facts blindly or at random.

This scheme would stimulate the student of criminology in his specialized researches, to broaden out the mental elaboration of his facts, correlating their values with other departments of science, because his guiding principles drawn from another field have to be continually in mind. He will be compelled, therefore, to use analogy and comprehensive comparisons. He must all the time compare the less pronounced phases of the functional mental phenomena in the diseased or defective representatives of the criminal classes with the more outspoken stadia *along the whole pathway of abnormal mental life.* It is particularly necessary that the study of the psychopathic or neuropathic criminal be made one of the integral parts in the organic whole of a coalition of sciences—psychiatric and neurological research. This is the most favorable standpoint for criminal anthropology to conduct its researches and make advances.

In regard to the physical variations in the criminal, we might proceed in the same way as in the investigation of the mental variations, that is, it will be necessary to have some principle to start with; some preliminary guiding idea as a groundwork for the collection and arrangement of the facts of the physical variation in the defective or diseased criminal.

Very little, if any good, can be gained by simply investigating these variations *en masse*, in the way one would use a net to entrap anything that comes in its way. The statistical elaboration of human physical variations *en masse* is liable to be of no use to the investigator himself or to others armed with some working hypothesis of variation and heredity. If the study of the variations is guided by some theory of the general operations of variation, even if the theory be faulty the facts will stand a better likelihood of being available, if not at present, at least in the future, as the general study of evolution finds more and more adequate theories.

One is not to collect, elaborate and make averages of measurements of so many hundreds or thousands of criminals because it may have happened that someone else has made a fewer number of measurements or by a different method, or because it seems a golden opportunity to fill up some minute crevice in anatomical observations. These things should be done with the distinct purpose of *solving some problem in man's biological relations*, and the statement of the problem should be deliberately formulated beforehand. To formulate the problem before beginning the observations brings out the all-important *motive* of the investigation. This motive is the guidance of the observations from a general study of heredity and variation and the states and value of the various working hypotheses of these two subjects. Without the motive the investigator lacks discipline and runs great risk of going astray and getting completely confused amid the facts collected.

How shall one find a guiding theory for the co-ordination of these physical variations among the defective or diseased criminals? By confining himself to the criminal alone, it is certainly hopeless to find any guiding principle. The facts of variations in man are indeed unique and highly valuable. Galton, the pioneer in the study of human heredity and variations, has reached many conclusions agreeing with many points worked out independently by Weismann, notably in the continuity of the germ plasm and the weak influence worked on it by the individual. But notwithstanding Galton's brilliant work anthropological studies in man alone have and can never form but an iota of the great drama of evolution, heredity and variation. Neither man nor any other living thing is intelligible if taken by itself. The phenomena of the whole organic realm are so interwoven that they must be surveyed throughout the whole series. Thus the study of variations and heredity involves the work in botany, zoology, paleontology and embryology, physiological as well as morphological. If, therefore, one would study intelligently the physical variations of the diseased or defective portions of the criminal classes, he must prepare for his work by gaining some general knowledge of evolution and variation and from this select his guiding principles for the formation of his facts. A difficulty arises immediately, for none of the theories of variation and heredity are at all adequate. Prof. Osborne points out the fact that the trend of study of evolution and heredity is now seeking a more well defined inductive and experimental basis. And with this established, the unknown factors in evolution may be brought to light, more probably through the labors of physiology than of pure morphology.

The questions in evolution have been stated rather than answered, and, as Osborne says, "we are entering the threshold of the evolution problem instead of standing within the portals. The hardest tasks lie before us, not behind us, and their solution will carry us well into the twentieth century."

The differentiation of palingenic from cenogenic variations, *of the time when a variation arises in the life-history of individual*, whether in gonagenic, gamogenic, embryogenic or somatogenic periods, and the investigation of the relations of the ontogenetic to phylogenetic variations are all factors of fundamental importance and cannot be cast aside in study of the human variations in anthropological investigation of the criminal or other defective classes. In short, he who would pursue the subject of the physical variations of the defective and diseased portions of the criminal classes must be a student of evolution and heredity.

And despite the excessive complications of the study of evolution and the wide range of its inquiry and the inadequate state of our knowledge, he must seek some guiding standpoint from the present working hypotheses in evolution at large, and proceed from it deductively in the study of pathological elements of the criminal classes. In this way even if the hypothesis has to be abandoned or modified in the future, the facts have been marshalled in an orderly way and are of service for re-elaboration, when the working theory becomes perfected. Difficult and comprehensive as is the study of variations in man in a certain small fraction of the race as in the criminal or defective classes, we may, nevertheless, hope that in the course of the deductive application of some working theory gathered from the general stock of knowledge of evolution some light will be reflected back on the general stock of our knowledge. The greater the number of standpoints sought after, the greater will be the progress, provided there is co-ordination with the diverging lines of other sciences.

While the great length of time elapsing in rendering a progressive variation continuous, is exceedingly discouraging and makes steady research in a particular instance well nigh impossible, there are opportunities for studies in man which, although limited, are nevertheless quite unique. We have in the first place the influence of experiment on the subject of ontogenetic variations and their relations to phylogenetic variations. I do not mean experiments such as can be devised and controlled by the investigator, but such as are already performed for him, by disease processes. These are in every sense of the word experiments of the most beautiful and ingenious kinds—nature's experiments. In the analysis of the several stages of formation of ontogenetic variations there certainly ought to be fine opportunities of research in the action of toxic agents, or other pathogenic stimuli (also defective cell food supplies) on the gonagenic variations as well as on the variations arising during the several periods of embryonic development. The phenomena of immunity, predisposition and vulnerability, inherited immunity, immunity as racial features ought to be most attractive fields for the general student of evolution. Furthermore, in man the opportunity is favorable for the study of repetition phenomena or reversion phenomena as possibly in the degenerative classes in idiocy, cretinism and epilepsy. There ought also to be in man material for attention to the dependence of ontogenetic *repetition* upon repetition in the environment and life habit, in contrast to the connection of ontogenetic *variation* with variation in environment and life habit. Particularly valuable would be the study of generations of delinquents in families, as in the remarkable investigations of the Jukes family.

The prison often contains inmates fit to be patients in the psychopathic hospital. Quite likely the psychopathic processes and certain portions of the criminal classes may reveal the initial stages of the process of neuron energy liberation, only here the process is spread out through a greater length of time. The ebb of neuron energy may have occurred through generations, and the neurasthenic phenomena concomitant with unloosening of the highest constellations of neurons having to do with inhibition, and the duties of *morale* and the guardianship of the finest and noblest of human emotions may occur most insidiously. The expenditure of neuron energy sinking in the course of many generations by almost infinitesimal and unnoticeable descents over the restitution-ascents of energy,* the higher neuron constellations in some particular man in a series of generations may utterly fail to develop the mechanism for elaboration of energy. Hence their parallel powers

* See paper on "Neuron Energy."

will be utterly lacking. Such a man may have no sense of morality and discipline and his subconscious self may tend to come out in all its nakedness.

I am not intimating here a transmission of acquired characteristics, that is that the receding tide of neuron energy in any individual influences the germ plasm to any extent. The external causes that liberate neuron energy in the individual affect the germ plasm simultaneously. These causes operating first in the highest and most unstable neuron may, to some slight extent, operate on the germ plasm in a secondary way from the damage to the neuron constellations. For these being progressively impaired both in extent and degree by the continuance of the external causes the general body forces (circulation, general metabolism in cellular food supply) may fall below par, and in this way exert a modifying influence on the germ plasm. But I prefer to think that the changes in the germ plasm passing on the continuance or preparation for the neurasthenia of the next generation are directly due to the same external causes such as toxic agents, deficient food supply to neuron that will bring about an undue liberation of neuron energy. The changes in the germ plasm are less dependent on the pathological expenditure of higher neuron energy than on the action of the same causes that also affect the neuron.

It seems to me that there are points of similarity between ordinary neurasthenia and the psychopathic conditions of certain criminal classes. And I think we may take it for granted that observation shows that some of the criminals certainly show psychopathic and even neuropathic phenomena. If we conceive that the ordinary type of the neurasthenic phase of the psychopathic process be stretched out through a greater space of time, so that it is exceedingly chronic and insidious, we have a mental picture of what may be taking place in the psychopathic criminal and what leads him to do his acts. This is not a mere speculation, for it is based on the general theory of neuron energy alluded to previously, derived from a certain range of facts forming a supporting groundwork. It is not at all difficult to conceive of the neurasthenic manifestations and their concomitant phases of the underlying pathological process as being more spread out in space and time (through members of generations) than we ordinarily witness in the symptoms in the concentrated phenomena in the ordinary form, occurring as an attack in a part of the life-history of the individual.

I am far, however, from making any sweeping application of the psychopathic basis of criminal acts, for who is to pronounce judgment upon right and wrong, or to give a standard of goodness in mankind? We can only look at the extremes, more or less, in delinquent actions. It seems best to seek out the more outspoken psychopathic cases in the prisons, and investigate them as comprehensively as possible, under the guidance of the neuron energy theory. The factor of environment is, of course, included in the study of the criminal in speaking of the guidance of the investigation from the standpoint of evolution. Anthropological investigation of this kind of the criminal, of the delinquent and defective classes may possibly prove valuable and fruitful. "Pathological anthropology," (by this I understand the study of human variations from the basis of pathology) is especially dependent for its success on a correlation of sciences after some such plan as we have endeavored to outline for psychiatric research. It is hard to see how anthropological investigations of this special kind can make any headway.

In centres of psychiatric research, criminal anthropology comes prominently to the surface in the direct and specialized investigation of the insane. For many systems of caring for the insane have to take into consideration the criminal insane and the insane criminal. In our own system, for instance, there is one special hospital set apart for the criminal insane. Here is a most valuable opportunity for getting at the borderland between the psychopathic criminal and the insane classes. Here is a class where the descending process of neuron energy liberation is outspoken and comes obtrusively to the surface. From this pivotal point the investigation should work in two directions: upward along the psychopathic channel toward the initial stages where the process approaches normal mental life, and downward in the abnormal mental life into deeper and deeper levels of insanity, both neuropathic and organic.

It seems to me that the hospital for the criminal insane offers the most absorbing and fruitful field of work for the anthropological psychiatrist. The differentiation between the criminal insane and the insane criminal seems to hinge upon a very insecure scientific basis. It is simply a question as to when the insanity was detected; if the individual committed a crime and there is insanity detected he is an insane criminal; if his insanity is first detected and then the crime is committed, he is a criminal insane. Both are of the same order, and their difference simply depends on the thoroughness of the examination. This distinction is therefore an arbitrary one. Further researches are greatly needed in the criminals exhibiting psychopathic phenomena. The diseased or defective criminal should be studied by the methods of psychology and psychopathology.

In regard to the inter-relation of the abnormal mental phenomena or mental variations with the physical variations, caution must be used lest one stumbles into pitfalls of error, and allows the fallacies of the simple method of enumeration to insinuate themselves into the elaboration of the facts. If one starts out with the idea that the mental departures in the criminal are in some way linked with the physical variations, both operative from a common cause or set of causes, it becomes easy to support the idea by collecting the instances which support the theory, and overlooking those which contradict it.

In statistical elaborations especially, this tendency to a greater or less degree, is often prone to occur. Among a large body of criminals the relation of physical variations to initial psychopathic phases might gain undue weight, unless we ascertain how far possibly the same set of variations may also occur in non-criminal classes, not associated with any psychopathic taint.

It might seem theorizing in advance of the facts that errors in the molecular structure of the germ plasm would first tell on the most supremely organized parts of the body (the highest congeries of the neuron constellations in the frontal lobes) without showing defects elsewhere in the body. It would seem that defects in the highest parts of the nervous system might occur without corresponding defects in the body. Conversely morphological defects in the body of any considerable degree would connote defective brain development. Facts show, however, that this may or may not be the case. Féré * has shown experimentally, that certain influences (noxious vapors,

* Bulletin de la Société de Biologie, 1896, p. 790.

mechanical vibrations) harmful to development if applied in a certain degree, may be favorable when applied in a lesser degree. Thus it seems that agents capable of exerting an influence resulting in an arrest of growth in one part may in the total development produce a superior individual. What is a drawback in one part may be a gain to another. Thus, some individuals with partial defects, have a remarkable general constitution. Hence, one often sees great minds dwelling in frail or ill-formed bodies. On the other hand, the agencies which we may imagine of a kind similar to those studied by Féré experimentally in the egg, may be of such a degree of intensity (auto-intoxications of the pregnant mother, other toxic and pathogenic agents and disturbances in the cellular food supply brought to bear from the mother to the fœtus) as to cause retardation of development without compensation in the nervous system or elsewhere. In this way weak individuals would be born without any saving graces. According to these experiments the matter hinges on the intensity of external agents.

Féré notes in harmony with his line of thought that the most civilized nations are distinguished by the number of extremes and exceptional beings: men of exceptional mental power, geniuses, and others intellectually and morally pervert. These latter are so because of deficient energy of the highest spheres of the brain unveiling in periods of time spread through a single individual or throughout generations the subconscious self which Sidis characterizes as "cowardly, brutal, credulous, suggestible, and devoid of all morality and conscience." These variations discussed by Féré, however, are to be carefully distinguished from the reversions or repetitions of variations. The interrelations of the physical and mental variations are enormously complex, but with what is known of the laws of mental life, heredity, and variations, or with such approaches as have been made toward these laws by psychology and the study of evolution to guide the research, we shall go less far astray by restricting the investigation to the criminal and endeavoring to find guiding theories in the restricted sphere of criminal anthropology alone.

It is somewhat customary in examining from time to time the status of a science and regarding its future progress, to look back into its past history and to go out of one's way by quoting selected passages from older observers, to show that they had premonitions of the knowledge of the present day. These retrospects are exceedingly interesting, but in most cases they are hardly worth the while, for in the past fifty years in many sciences the knowledge is quite divergent, and indeed is often totally different from that of the preceding periods. The reason is, the methods of investigation are now totally different; they are more exact and of more extensive scope. The past of criminal anthropology is interesting, however, for it shows that the subject is worthy of a division of labor in the community of sciences, and should be given the attention of a distinct science of its own. There has been a steady growth leading up to the formation of the science of criminal anthropology and its pedigree is quite old.

Plato and Aristotle made studies of physiognomy and attempted to work out the physical and psychological correspondence of the passions of men and their facial expressions. From these early studies to comparatively recent times there have been numerous attempts to establish a relation between certain physical (anatomical) conditions and abnormal psychical states. As a result, however, of the isolation of these investigators and their dependence on speculations in lieu of adequate methods of studying facts their studies present much repetition and consequently useless work. Notwithstanding this it is possible to trace in these and later works a gradual growth and a steady advancement which forms the basis of our present view of the unstable classes. Upon these works criminal anthropology was founded.

The study of the criminal has not leaped into a sudden or distrustful existence, but has behind it the momentum of centuries of thought along the idea of the linking of man's physical and mental variations. The study of physiognomy was revived by the Jesuit Niquetius, by Cortes, Candamus, De la Chambre, Della Porta, etc., who were the precursors of Gall, Spurzheim and Levator on the one hand, and on the other of the modern scientific study of the emotions with their expressions, in face and gesture, conducted by Camper, Bell, Engle, Schaffhausen, Schack, Heiment, and above all by Darwin. Gall's theories were applied in the examinations of criminals by Lauvergne (1841) and Attomyr (1842), but they carried the figments of phrenology to the extreme. DeRolandes (Italy, 1835) published observations on a deceased criminal; Sampson (America, 1846) tried to trace the connection of criminal phenomena and cerebral organization; Camper (Germany, 1854) published a study on the physiognomy of murderers, and Lallement (1858–1862) published a long work on criminals from a psychological point of view. The science of criminal anthropology, strictly speaking, only began with Forbes Winslow (1854), Mayherr (1860), Thompson (1870), Wilson (1870), Nicolson, Maudsley (1873) and the notable observations of Despine (1868) and finally of Lombroso.

Since 1876 a number of writers have published valuable additional studies of the criminal, and have established the fact that indications of psychopathic and neuropathic processes frequently appear in individual members of this class. Experience also demonstrates that quite a share of crimes are committed by persons who are insane in the ordinary acceptance of the word, or at least who may be said to have the prodromata of insanity. In addition to the prison we have in mind the extension of anthropological work in the reformatories among the refractory and delinquent juveniles, the epileptics, the deaf and dumb, and the blind, or secure co-operation in work from those having charge of these classes. Among the idiots the work ought also to be very promising, and throw light upon the *modus operandi* of this effect, and especially upon their classification, unless this has been worked out satisfactorily by such investigators as Sollier, Petersen and Ireland. One quite certain indication of the increasing momentum of the study of criminology and allied subjects is the appearance of special journals on the subject. Germany and Italy each have a journal for the dissemination of the accumulating knowledge on this subject.

The great difficulty encountered in this investigation is the selection of a normal standard whereby to measure the abnormal departure. In this country where the population is so hetergeneous, we are immediately confronted by the difficulty of finding a standard race type to measure by, and in fact we can find no absolute standard. Only a standard varying between certain small limits can be used. We also hope by means of this department of anthropology to study the phenomena of deterioration in the criminal and in the epileptic.

Immediate results can hardly be expected from this department. The amount of work falling within the scope of anthropological investigations of the early phases of insanity is stupendous. It can only be done little by little, and must grow and develop in the course of years. Any work along these lines such as previously indicated, to be of any value whatsoever, must be most carefully planned. It cannot be forced along with undue haste. One must, therefore, ask patience in expectation of results from this branch of investigation, the more so, since there is no well defined and no established precedent to follow. The work is of a pioneer character, and this as a rule meets with failures, and often has to begin over again, profiting by its mistakes, and has frequently to readjust its plan and methods of work. From time to time results may be published as to the progress of this department, but they cannot be had all at once.

A very interesting piece of work now in progress in the department of anthropology is a study of the correlation of the mental and physical growth of some young boys in a disciplinarian school. This has been undertaken in conjunction with Doctor Downing, of Brooklyn, N. Y. Fortunately we have an opportunity of studying these boys for several years, in order that we may fully record the relationship of psychical and physical growth, and also identify those among them who tend to deflect into the pathway of degeneracy. In short, the main object of the department of anthropology is to identify and study by means of scientific methods the degenerate, the candidates for the prison, the reformatory and asylums. It must be seen how important is some attempt at gaining a coherent knowledge of the insane before they make their way into the hospitals. When this is known, it is bound to be of practical benefit and yield economical returns by instituting some form of control of insanity before it reaches its more hopeless stages.

In brief, one prominent purpose of anthropology at the Institute is to ascertain the proportion of cases of insanity occurring in normal individuals, in individuals who have no hereditary predisposition toward insanity—and to compare this proportion with the other cases of insanity complicated with or resulting from hereditary predisposition. For in the former class of cases insanity is more or less of an accident, and in the great majority of cases recovery is to be expected; whereas in the latter class with predisposition recovery is much less liable to occur. The determination of this question is most important.

The instruments required for this department are comparatively simple and inexpensive. It has apparatus for testing the acuteness of the senses and sundry instruments for physical measurements of the human body; two instruments to measure the diameter and contour of the skull, one in duplicate for the use of the State hospitals; measures for determining the cubic contents of the skull; a stereograph for tracing contours and profiles of the skull, and an anthropometer used for taking general measurements of the body.

We hope in the course of time to make a collection of skeletons of the insane, in order to study the stigmata of degeneracy in the osseous system. These skeletons can be exhumed without much expense, after the cadaver has remained in suitable soil for two or three years.

The anthropological institute at Paris is very proud of

the collection of the complete skeletons of thirteen epileptics, because their histories and behavior during life are accurately known. Seeing that the histories of our patients at the hospitals are scrupulously kept, we ought to be able in the course of time to have one of the best collections in the world for studying the osseous systems of epileptics, criminals and lunatics. The value of this collection does not lie in the fact that it is a mere conglomeration of bones, but that it should be possible to study each skeleton in connection with the life-history of its possessor.

The department is in charge of Alois Hrdlicka, M. D.

Chapter XIII.

THE UNCLASSIFIED RESIDUUM.

In concluding these remarks on the correlation of several branches of scientific research in the investigation of the life-history of insanity,* a paragraph from one of Professor James' essays† is most appropriate.

"The great field for new discoveries," said a scientific friend to me the other day, "is always the unclassified residuum. Round about the accredited and orderly facts of every science there ever floats a sort of dust cloud of exceptional observations, of occurrences minute and irreg-

* It should not be considered that a centre of psychiatric study, such as the Pathological Institute of the New York State Hospitals, has overreached itself in bringing unnecessary or irrelevant departments of science to bear upon the problems of psychopathology and psychiatry, or that in taking a stand against the restricted study of insanity it has gone to the opposite extreme in too greatly diversifying this research. The fact that there is no assistant in psychology and psychopathology, that there is but one associate for the whole comprehensive department of pathological anatomy, and that there is no representative for the department of normal histology of the nervous system nor for experimental pathology and hæmatology, shows that this projected plan of the correlation of branches of scientific research in insanity at this Institute is still not completely developed.

† "The Will to Believe and other Essays in Popular Philosophy," p. 299.

ular and seldom met with, which it always proves more easy to ignore than to attend to. The ideal of every science is that of a closed and completed system of truth. The charm of most sciences to their more passive disciples consists in their appearing, in fact, to wear just this ideal form. Each one of our various *ologies* seems to offer a definite head of classification for every possible phenomenon which it professes to cover; and so far from free is most men's fancy, that, when a consistent and organized scheme of this sort has once been comprehended and assimilated, a different scheme is unimaginable. No alternative, whether to whole or parts, can any longer be conceived as possible. Phenomena unclassifiable within the system are therefore paradoxical absurdities, and must be held untrue. When, moreover, as so often happens, the reports of them are vague and indirect; whether they come as mere marvels and oddities rather than things of serious moment—one neglects or denies them with the best of scientific consciences. Only the born geniuses let themselves be worried and fascinated by these outstanding exceptions and get no peace until they are brought within the fold. Your Galileos, Galvanis, Fresnels, Purkinjes, and Darwins are always getting confounded and troubled by insignificant things. Any one will renovate his science who will steadily look after the irregular phenomena. And when science is renewed, its new formulas often have more of the voice of the exceptions in them than that of what were supposed to be the rules."

Surely from the scientific standpoint the disordered states of consciousness in insanity form a very large "unclassified residuum." In correlating the branches of sciences we have avoided the danger indicated by Professor James, namely, the restriction of a branch of science to some fixed and narrow limits of observation. If a branch of science be thus restricted it soon becomes walled up within itself. It travels in a rut, repeats its old observations over and over again, trying to make them appear new by merely setting them forth in new words, or what is still more deceptive, marshalling and exhibiting them in diversely colored plates of differently stained sections; it finally becomes worn out and mummified. On the other hand, if a branch of science seems to be nearing the limits of its capacity to formulate new generalizations, when it seems to have completed its possible activities in presenting the ideal "closed system" of truths to which there seems nothing to add, such a science, when extended to the outlying domain intervening between a sister science, may have to begin its investigations all over again in a new and broader light. *Modern specialization among the branches of science is creating gaps and clefts which contain more important fields for investigation than the individual departments of science themselves.* He who can bridge over the rifts between the border lines of several of these sciences will discover the richest domains of investigation and gather in a good harvest of scientific truths. *It is the value of the domains between the various medical and biological "ologies," when guided by psychology and psychopathology that we have endeavored to bring into prominence in the study of insanity.*

Chapter XIV.

THE FUTURE OF PSYCHIATRY.

We have pointed out some of the natural shortcomings of psychiatry, inevitable in the evolution of its progress; we must now behold the greatness of its future. It would be a carping and disrespectful form of scientific *lèse majesté* to point out the shortcomings of psychiatry as a stigma on the name of the science, for it is truly destined to be the most majestic of all the biological and medical sciences.

The shortcomings of psychiatry only serve to show the greatness, comprehensiveness and difficulties of the science. The other sciences in medicine and biology are elementary beside psychiatry. They are but stepping-stones to psychiatry and psychology. For the two are synonymous in studying the abnormal phenomena of consciousness. Psychiatry should never be so narrowly viewed as being tied down only to insanity, it also deals with abnormal phenomena of consciousness in general, the domain of psychopathology. The study of abnormal manifestations of consciousness presupposes some knowledge of normal psychology while at the same time it is the only key to an understanding of normal mental phenomena.

It is not strange that psychiatry, the most difficult and comprehensive of all medical and biological sciences, has been one of the last to begin its scientific progress. Psychiatry has not lagged behind of its own accord; it has been held back and had no choice but to wait until its stepping-stones might be built. It has had to wait for the growth of psychology in general and psychopathology in particular; it has had to wait for cellular biology, pathological anatomy, neural anatomy, and their affiliated branches of research to attain sufficient development to cope with the difficult problems of psychiatry. Psychiatry for the short history of its existence has done its utmost with the imperfect methods at its disposal, and is now looking for new methods to fertilize its soil, highly fruitful, but difficult to till. When it is perceived how far the subsidiary sciences have had to develop before attaining the capacity to be of service to psychiatry, we can gain some idea of the eminence of psychiatry among the medico-biological sciences.

Psychology, psychopathology and psychiatry are destined to form the loftiest pinnacle of the temple of science. The scientific story of the rocks holds one spell-bound; the history of the egg or the mechanism of a tiny organism have their fascination; mathematics and the laws which command the courses of the stars are awe-inspiring, but none of these sciences or their allies have the grandeur or are so deeply and essentially human as the three sciences—psychology, psychopathology and psychiatry—for they unveil the greatest marvel of the universe—the human mind. Well may we say with the great Scotch philosopher: "In the world there is nothing greater than man, and in man there is nothing greater than mind." A knowledge of mind, both in its normal and abnormal manifestations, is the science of sciences.

The common run of neurologists and pathologists, in their mistaken nature of the true function of science, lose more and more sight of what lies beyond their microscopic field of vision. What is still sadder, they are absurdly proud of their narrowness, making a virtue of their shortcomings; their ignorance is as great as their conceit is infinite. They highly value the process of groping aimlessly in the dark for new details. All explanation, all rational interpretation, is shunned as a pest, and under the stigma of "theory" is kept in abhorrence; all comprehension of phenomena, all generalization, is branded by the name of "metaphysics" and is sneered at, and ridiculed, and held in contempt. The more meaningless, the more inexplicable a detail is, the more is it treasured and valued as a "good fact" purified of all extraneous dross, such as reason and understanding, which are branded as a vice, as "theory and metaphysics." And yet these very neurologists, histologists and pathologists who suffer from intellectual photophobia or phrenophobia are the worst type of dogmatists, the least intelligent class of unconscious metaphysicians, inasmuch as they revere only the chaotic, the irrational and the incomprehensible. It is only the best thinking men among them who begin to look for light and for a broad horizon. The psychiatrist, on the contrary, by the very nature of his studies, is forced more and more to broaden out the basis of his science. Nothing short *of a co-operation of all the medico-biological and psychological sciences* is what psychiatry requires. The enlightened psychiatrist looks for an *organization* of the dispersed and dismembered parts of medical science. Medicine has usurped the psychological guidance of psychiatry altogether too long.

Fortunately this enlightened spirit found a foothold in the Commission and the representatives of the New York State Hospitals, and for the first time in the history of science was an Institute established on a broad scientific basis, an Institute whose aim is to till the field of psychiatry by means of instruments and methods obtained through an organized federation of the most important and most vital branches of biological and psychological sciences. Such a federation is not only indispensable to the growth of psychiatry, but is also most essential to the development of biology, psychology and exact medical knowledge in general. Men of science ought to be grateful to the psychiatrist for the mere fact that he is the first to call for a *general unified* activity of many branches of science. For *unification* means *generalization*, the discovery of *laws*, the true aim of science.

PART III.

Chapter XV.

FACTS AND THEORIES IN MEDICAL SCIENCE.

When a scientist ventures into foreign fields, he can return to his own particular territory with new and broader ideas and recast his whole trend of observation; he becomes possessed of the power of larger guiding principles; he has the great advantage of guiding his work with discrimination and of seeing what is essential, passing by what is accessory; he sees better through the relation and interdependence of things instead of trying to hit upon them by shuffling the facts about; he has a discontent with the scope of his former work and seeks to look further beyond the proximate into the remote. Such a spirit of discontent is the watchword of progress in science.

Meanwhile the venturesome traveler must expect distrust from those who are working in these other fields; for both they and he know that only the crust and the surface are being inspected by the outsider who can have no grasp of the depths and the details. On the other hand, he must also expect to be openly or secretly discredited by his colleagues who remain at home quietly working out their results, and must also expect to be looked upon as having fallen behind in the ranks, because he left the work desk and the machinery idle for the sake of reflection. He is liable also to fall under the stigma of having been affected by unsound ideas; and although this should entail caution, it is not to be held in excessive apprehension. Altogether the task of broad generalization and correlation is not inviting, and, besides, the great labor, the distrust and opposition met with, make one averse to undertake such a work. If the journey be at all extensive, it will indeed be strange, if one does not return with a burdensome sense of oppression at the vastness of what lies before him in other strange pathways. The pioneer in science may feel like Humboldt bewildered at the fathomless depths of nature, not knowing where to pick up the guiding threads for explanation.

In this cursory glimpse of a few departments one cannot help feeling great dissatisfaction with the way the subject of the importance and value of correlation in psychiatry has been presented. Many points of importance have been barely touched upon and others have been entirely omitted. Yet no such vast plan was ever entertained of attempting a comprehensive sweep of so many sciences. The attitude has been to look at the borderlands of the branches of research, to glance at their confines and at their points of coalescence, and from this to gather ideas, guiding principles and methods whereby psychiatry might open a new pathway. With some key, some broad idea derived from a study of consciousness and fortified by some psycho-physiological principle, we work deductively and use the phenomena in psychiatry for verification. In this deductive process these several sciences would also be of use in the verification in their several bearings on abnormal mental life and also reflect light on the theory from an inductive standpoint.

A thing that has augmented the dissatisfaction with this writing almost to the point of discouragement is that certain matters have been accorded a prominence and emphasis which in a little while will surely seem obvious. It may be, however, that what seems exceedingly elementary in some places, as befits a discussion of this character, is somewhat balanced by being interwoven in other places with ideas that are not wholly superficial. I think also that in a little while they who secretly and openly discredit such an ideal, because it has not fallen into the conventional and hopeless groove, will be the very ones to take the whole plan of the correlation of sciences in psychiatry for granted, as an indispensable and obvious means of progress, as is usually the case with all departures from the beaten track. Yet at this particular time one finds it necessary, elementary though as it will appear a few years later, to defend the use of the several branches of research in their correlation and organization for the benefit of psychiatry.

One may get suggestions of deep application and pivotal points to work out brilliant theories in disease process by reflecting on the analogy of the human commonwealth of cells with the social organism. Take out the factor of correlation and interdependence of the parts, and progress stops—the organism, social, living or scientific, falls to pieces. Restrict psychiatry to the microscope, and it is impossible to gain the momentum and power of the correlated sciences—aside from the fact that from the very nature of microscopic research, it is not even on the right road to solve the problems of abnormal mental life.

At one moment psychiatry is taken to task, because it does not progress, at the next moment, because it does attempt progress. The attitude is absurd, yet unfortunately on the ground of expediency, it is also to be feared. It is to be feared, because it measures the work of an institution of this kind by the false standard of simple mechanical fact-gathering mainly through pathological anatomy. This is unfortunate, but it cannot stay the progress of psychiatry. Progress in psychiatry is bound to come, it is inevitable.

There is a great difference between "work in science" and "scientific work." In "work in science" mechanical work is at a maximum, and reasoning at a minimum; in "scientific work" the reverse is the case. Shall work in pathological anatomy and bacteriology remain the main avenue of scientific psychiatric research? Shall we have men satisfied with the act of pouring forth into the already swollen streams of literature desultory microscopical details, the real task, the true aim of science, being left undone? Is there not already enough of such work, in medicine, or is the work to create what might seem an admirable spirit of emulation by detailed description of minuteness outdoing the devils of whom it is said that some twenty thousand can dance on the point of a needle without causing the least friction? We do not get explanation by miniaturing the problem. If the microscope could get down to still smaller particles the same old question is still on hand, as to why the particles dance and what makes them dance.

What becomes of many of such descriptions after they are discharged into medical or psychiatric literature? After the first ephemeral notice is passed, they are shelved with the rest of the lumber to be dusted off occasionally, when someone else on a like errand compares them with his own results showing wherein he agrees and also wherein he disagrees. The title of the work also adorns its appropriate line in the bibliographical annex of other papers.

When the collection of facts is to be made use of, observe what is done by the man of ideas. He quietly appropriates the work and puts a value on it. Armed with a play of the imagination, he makes a mental elaboration of the facts; interweaves them with theory.

Meanwhile from the men of facts a storm of disapproval comes. They are grieved, because they think they have done the real hard work and a marauding theorist has plundered them of it. What aggravates the matter is that the man of ideas seems gifted with a strange and vexatious ingenuity of eliciting what he can make use of, what fits in and dovetails with his ideas.

Often, however, perhaps as a rule, the desultory "new" facts collected by the "workers" remain in their chaotic and worthless state,—they cannot be utilized by the man who works from the standpoint of ideas and theories. This is because when facts are described and catalogued by the workers, that which is frivolous, inconsequential, and accessory, is given just as much weight as that which is essential and of pivotal value to test a theory. The worker cannot separate the indifferent from the essential. How can he appreciate the essential without knowing what he is striving after or not having any idea of what he wants to prove and solve? In pathological anatomy, for example, is there not amid the plenty of facts a dearth of ideas? Do we gain, for instance, anything by saying that in hyperplasia the tissue grows, because the inhibition to growth is removed? This subterfuge does not explain anything. And yet the phenomenon has a deep significance when its explanation is realized in the light of a broad range of thought.

The students of pathological anatomy make a mistake in studying man by himself and as a species discontinuous from other forms of life. The study of an animal is not intelligible when the animal is taken by itself, away from its environment, out of its place in the whole range of animal life. If medical men have fallen into the habit of believing that the microscope is the guide to medical science and that pathological anatomy is the great and main line of investigation, must psychiatry also follow suit, or rather, remain in the same rut? If in medicine the idea is prevalent that descriptions of the facts of abnormal structure accomplish the main aim of scientific research, must psychiatric study be discouraged, because it would abandon this delusion? In science the influence of the beaten track must not arbitrarily repress that which departs from it.

It is very sad to find that some medical men, men who ought to know better, are under the delusion, prevalent only among the least educated classes of the profession, that the main point of science in general consists in recording facts in pathological anatomy and bacteriology. The same thing is expected of psychiatry and all original research work that does not follow the beaten track of medical science is abused and decried. But how will the advance of psychiatry be attained by recording facts in pathological anatomy? To attempt to make the study of pathological anatomy the guiding motive of research in the phenomena of abnormal mental life is a snare and delusion, sheer folly.

The demand to throw out on the would-be scientific market a mass of incoherent facts, as if it were accomplishing the real work of science, is unreasonable. Dumping facts into so-called scientific medical literature would have been an easy and simple matter. Indeed, a great number of facts have been gathered at the Institute by a great variety of methods. The brain has been thrust into the crucible and its ashes determined, it has been rended with acids and alkalies, it has been preserved in many fluids and stained with many dyes, giving rise to many plates with diversity of color; guinea pigs, monkeys and rabbits have had their share of toxines and bacteria; in fact it appears that the particular demon presiding over a certain form of meningitis has been caught, registered, put in the culture tube, and given a proper place among his associates in the bacteriological collection. Yet how does the mere statement of all these facts in any way explain the phenomena of insanity? Which is it best to do? Pour out these facts into the literature just as they are found, or attempt to co-ordinate, arrange them in harmony with theory, and endeavor to see their relation to the problems of abnormal mental life? We have endeavored to maintain a higher ideal than to record facts blindly.

The aim of this Institute is not to collect blindly and irrationally masses of incoherent facts and of confused new details, the cherished ideal of the school or rather of the crowd of the so-called scientific "workers." The Institute is a scientific centre and as such it aims to cultivate science in a rational way making use of inductive and deductive methods, guided by theory, hypothesis and speculation; it works at facts in order to solve a problem, in order to make use of the facts and not merely to collect them without separating the chaff from the kernel. The facts collected, whether of our finding or discovered by others, are as far as possible governed by guiding principles, broad theories, theories consistent with the body of knowledge gained in other directions. If the study of facts is not guided in this way, it is hard to see, no matter how fine the details and how close the observation, how such blind recording of facts can possibly avoid confusion. On the other hand, one must fully understand the danger of ill-founded speculation, of speculation wrought out of a limited and specialized range of observation, of speculation announced without sufficient verification.

Some medical men have queer notions of the meaning of "work" in science. In all other walks of life work must have a definite purpose—only in science work should be done blindly, without any aim, work for the sake of the work itself. If in life we require understanding of the work and knowledge of its purpose, the purpose guiding the work, why should ignorance of purpose be considered a virtue in science? Are blindness and ignorance special attributes of medical science? Most certainly not.

In this age of feverish activity hundreds and hundreds of men are working in an almost delirious haste in laboratories scattered all over the civilized globe to obtain priority of recognition in the discovery of new facts. Great masses of desultory, fragmentary, inco-ordinated descriptions of facts are recorded in scores of specialized journals. Even in the same laboratory men are working side by side and still independently isolating their fields of inquiry. Their chief aim seems to be to find something that no one else has worked upon, in order that it may be *new*, however insignificant it may be otherwise. Most of all, instead of suspecting where to find the new facts by premeditation, they expect to hit on them by the doctrine of chance, by straining everything that comes along in their nets in the hope of finding something new that may be described. The chief ambition of these workers in science is to dump into the literature four or five times a year a mass of inco-ordinated facts. Surely it were better, if the energy expended in this haste and hurry of announcing and recording details were employed in co-ordinating the facts before publication.

In the midst of all this, is it not well to pause and reflect that in the feverish fact-collecting activity we run the risk of losing sight of the true aim of science? Students are too prone to take it for granted that the aim of science is fulfilled by the mechanical labor at the work desk and dexterity with technical methods; they are often absolutely innocent of the true aim of science, namely, generalization.

Science seems to be a race for new details, and when these are found the inquiry is at an end. Bacteriology has joined in the game with pathological anatomy, and the prize is given to the man who can catch a new devil, presiding in tutelary fashion over some disease entity, and bottle him up in the culture tube. To identify the proximate causes of disease is of enormous value from the standpoint of utility, but one must not deceive himself in thinking that this explains the process, the *modus operandi* of abnormal function.

Pathological anatomy has more need of new theories than of new facts. I hope this intimation that pathological anatomy is making the mistake of thinking that fact-gathering fulfills the true aim of science does not seem hasty, or reckless. Among the several branches of science reviewed, I feel less utterly confined to the surface of the inquiry of this department, and, thanks to my master, I have also had the opportunity of having some insight into its philosophy. Hence reflection over its deficiencies does not warp the vision of its strength, its scientific dignity, and its achievements. But these achievements must not blind us to the fact that science does not make progress by studying proximate causes only; nor are we to fall into the habit of believing that unreflective observation, no matter how close, or voluminous, fulfills the true purpose of science. There must also be the *reflective formulation* of the observations. To find truth, to discover law, thought and reflection must be used.

I do not mean to say that pathological anatomy has no

theories. It uses deduction in its own special line of inquiry; and this is just the trouble. The theories seem well grounded, if surveyed by the narrow extent of territory from which they are drawn, but when tested by a wider range of thought, they are inadequate and even absurd. The theories are derived from causes which lie too adjacent to the effects. Hence the pathological anatomist is continually turning out new facts which he cannot make use of.

Some of the pathological anatomists have not the first, most elementary notion of the purpose of science, namely—*generalization of facts and deduction of laws.* Many so-called scientists are only concerned with getting the facts catalogued. Pathological anatomy is in much the same condition that biology was before Darwin's time; like pre-Darwinian biology it consists of an appalling mass of facts, piled up by hundreds of men working in many independent, highly specialized fields, all striving to get hold of "something new." Instead of being properly co-ordinated before being published, all this is thrown into the literature just as it is fresh from the work desk. What a great opportunity it is for some one with grasp of mind to enter the field of pathological anatomy with a great general co-ordinating principle to unite these scattered facts and give them their appropriate theorectical valuation. Such a man can spare himself the trouble of delving out new facts. He may have to go, occasionally, to the laboratory desk, but then it will be with the distinct purpose of seeking some pivotal fact; some crucial experiment to test his theory.

The pathological anatomist has not only fallen into the mistake of thinking that his science consists of mere purposeless fact-gathering, but he is also leading general medicine astray. Pathological anatomy and especially bacteriology from their lack of broad theories, instead of correcting the mistake, have only helped to confirm general medical belief in the erroneous conception of the nature of disease. Diseases are looked upon as entities, individualities, specific things, each with its specific cause or set of causes. Contentment with this idea of the proximate cause of disease simply wards off inquiry for wider generalization of thought. The narrow views of pathological anatomy and bacteriology dominate too much the whole trend of scientific medical thought.

Pathological anatomy, setting too much store on the simple task of observing and gathering facts and too little on ascertaining their significance, and general medicine, looking too much to this branch as its guide, it would be strange, if medicine did not come to be more confirmed than ever to look upon this "collection" work as the true standard of scientific research. So indeed it has happened. In medicine it is taken for granted that all of its branches should conform to the same standard and conduct its researches after the example set by pathological anatomy. For pathological anatomy and bacteriology have done grand service for the art of medicine. It would also be strange, if under this medical conception of science, theory and speculation were not greatly distrusted. This is also the case. Attempts to theorize are not infrequently held up to ridicule and scorn and considered prejudicial to the advance of science. It is certainly unfortunate that in medicine art is guiding science.

We go on discouraging theory and speculation, and yet this is the soul of science and the mainspring of its progress. We go on warning each other against philosophy in science, yet without philosophy there is no science.

Johannes Müller says of physiology that without philosophy it is no science at all. We must, however, remember that men naturally fall into two classes. By far the greater number have minds that can only concern themselves with the adjacent and the proximate. The synthetic mind that looks above and beyond the immediate and the surface of things is unfortunately a rarity, a form of genius. We should encourage this form of genius and provide suitable environment that it may thrive. We go on discrediting those who come from foreign fields of research to work in our own particular territory, yet I think we ought to welcome these outsiders who come to look over our facts and take a comprehensive glance, perhaps, not a profound view of our work, as they are often better equipped to theorize over our facts than we who are deeply immersed in some fragmentary, dismembered part of our science.

Chapter XVI.

THE PATHO-ANATOMIST AND THE CLINICIAN.

The great science in medicine is general physiology and pathological physiology in particular. It is in biology, general physiology and psychopathology that the philosophy of medicine is to be sought. *Function presupposes structure.* If we would understand disease, we must naturally study the living phenomena. This the clinician does, and the scientific clinician is in fact a physiologist and psychopathologist, for he studies function. And he is in a far better position to perceive the great guiding principle—in the study of abnormal manifestations—the energy basis of function, than the observer with the microscope. The pathological physiologist, or, if you please, the clinician, perceives the actual manifestations and activities of the disease process, whereas the man with the microscope only sees the tracks of it, the footprints as it were. The one studies dynamics, the other the statics of disease. The study of the footprints of energy is valuable; it is a study of the effects of the process, but not of the process itself. If one would understand the footprints, he must also study the thing that made them.

The pathological anatomist often feels sorry for the clinician because the latter does not set much store by the "granules," yet it is interesting to watch the clinician use the microscope. He gains an idea from the observation of the living phenomena and uses the microscope with a distinct purpose, and as a means of verifying his idea and casting light on it. He seems quite indifferent to many ultra details of structure which the anatomist guards with great jealousy and the want of which is evidence of a lamentable lack of knowledge and held up as a warning against intrusion into a foreign precinct. But the clinician is like the physicist seeking to explain the activities of a mechanism, why and how it works, and what animates it. The color the mechanism is painted with, the oil spots, the dust marks and the like facts which the type of the mechanical, unreflective anatomist would lay equal stress with the other parts, the physicist cares very little about; what he wants to know is the general construction of the machine, and in explaining its working, he talks in the language of physics and in terms of energy.

When the scientific clinician finishes with the microscopic work, one is liable to find that it has contributed some explanation of the disease process, a thing so often left undone by the anatomist, because he cannot guide his work and fully understand the facts without a general knowledge of function and its relations to energy. Meanwhile, the anatomist observing the crudeness of the clinician's technical methods with the microscope (which, of course, is not to be commended), is inclined to think that the clinician's conclusions are erroneous, his views unsound, and are to be avoided. Yet the clinician endeavors to find the meaning of the lesion and of the disease process, and is in fact far more scientific than his friend the patho-anatomist.

Chapter XVII.

THE PATHOLOGICAL INSTITUTE AND PSYCHIATRY.

Pathological anatomy and bacteriology have an undue influence in moulding medical scientific thought and activity. This being the case medicine expects that scientific research in psychiatry should pursue the same channel, an absolutely profitless task. There is no use of deluding ourselves in the hope that we can make progress in the investigation of abnormal mental life under the guidance of pathological anatomy and bacteriology.

The finding of proximate causes does not explain insanity. I might as well say at once that this Institute was not built up on the plan of simply assembling these several branches of research and plunging into them blindly, describing facts without stopping to reflect on the general aim of the institution itself. Nor was it founded on the plan of using the mainstays of medical research, such as physiological chemistry, and particularly pathological anatomy, as the principal and guiding branches of research in psychiatry. Nor was it based on the plan of simply delving out any facts that research in these branches might unearth and expecting to hit, by happy chance, on some discovery of the *modus operandi* of abnormal mental life. No such plan was ever entertained.

The guidance of psychiatric research by the medical

conception of using anatomy, chemistry and bacteriology, would have been simple. We should merely have to follow the precedent of the pathological laboratory in medicine and extend it by adding chemistry and bacteriology. By focussing these sciences on autopsy material from the asylum or from hospitals of nervous diseases, recording the observations and then publishing them, side by side with the superficial clinical history, the task would have been finished and much "work" could have been put forth with that degree of celerity which the pressure for results demands from an institution of this kind before it can even become organized.

The medical conception of guiding psychiatric research by branches of investigation that do not in the least take account of the phenomena of mental life is utterly wrong. Had we, however, followed out this simple and fallacious plan of psychiatric investigation and poured forth observations of this character, it would have fulfilled the expectation of the medical conception of the research, met with approval, and the ordeal of trying to maintain a higher ideal could have been avoided. Meanwhile the psychiatrist, unless also influenced by the medical conception of the research, on observing this work might well remark: "This is the same old stuff only on a larger scale. The granules in the neuron are exceedingly fine and quite new. The chemical analyses of the excretions are more searching than formerly. The toxic factor in some forms of mental disease is more thoroughly verified. But through no stretch of sophistry am I able to find any approach to the explanation of the living phenomena—insanity itself. I still have no key to the solution of the general problem of abnormal mental life." On the other hand, if we adhere to the ideal of endeavoring to furnish explanations of abnormal mental life and abandon the medical conception of psychiatric research, we run the risk of losing favor with the medical "ologists," such as the neurologist, pathologist, histologist, bacteriologist, etc., and perhaps with some psychiatrists, who under the influence of their medical training take the same narrow and fallacious view of psychiatric research.

In the midst of these difficulties, however, the choice is definite and clear. We are to follow out the true aim of science and to work out explanations, *theories* and *generalizations* of the abnormal phenomena of consciousness. To do this we cannot use the medical branches of pathological anatomy, physiological chemistry and bacteriology as the guiding sciences in our ideal of psychiatric investigation. These branches must be made entirely *secondary* and *auxiliary* to *general physiology*, *psychopathology* and *psychology*. I sincerely hope that we shall not be misjudged, if we have not brought forth various inco-ordinate observations on the dead tissues of the insane along purely medical lines of investigation, as though this could furnish any key to the understanding of living phenomena of abnormal mental life. We have desired to avoid this kind of work, unless it could *subserve some purpose in the explanation of insanity*.

I think it must be quite plain that, if we would ever find any key to the explanation of insanity, we had best first and foremost investigate the living phenomena of insanity and not by sciences which have to do with the third and fourth degree concomitants of abnormal phenomena of consciousness, such as anatomy and chemistry. If we wish to understand the *modus operandi* of insanity, let us by all means go directly to the fountain-head and give up the hopeless task of inductive ascent from the far distant by-waters and remote side-channels of medical research. *We must study insanity itself,—we must examine, investigate and experiment on the living patient.*

Hitherto and even at the present time two obstacles have stood in the way of a direct psychopathological study of insanity. In the first place, a purely medical education does not only prepare one for the study of the abnormal phenomena of consciousness, but actually leads him astray. *Medical training leaves out psychology, the only science which can guide investigation of abnormal mental life,* and it is useless to try to substitute other sciences. In the second place, the difficulty of finding any well-grounded working hypothesis of insanity is further augmented by the fact that asylum cases are too advanced and far too greatly complicated to yield the key. What holds the science of psychiatry back is the fact of its being guided by medicine; it is a case of the blind leading the blind.

The plan of this Institute has been to make psychological groups of sciences the guide of psychiatric research. From the very beginning all our efforts were directed towards one aim,—the discovery of some general principle of abnormal mental life. The idea was to study the living phenomena of abnormal consciousness and find a working theory of the *modus operandi* of these phenomena. I think, if we wish to accomplish scientific work, the first thing to do is to survey the field by independent thought, and not be governed by too excessive a veneration for tradition, dogma and the formalism of the schools.

The first thing is to state the problem, to find out what is to be done. The second step is to find out how to solve the problem. The problem is the explanation of abnormal phenomena of consciousness, the discovery of their laws. The way to solve the problem is very obviously by means of the sciences of consciousness, namely, psychology and psychopathology—and by this means alone. Start with this idea and you will be able to estimate the proper value of the medical branches of research in relation to psychiatry, and know how to use them. *In psychiatric research, especially when a working hypothesis is absolutely indispensable, medical sciences are to take second and not first place.*

The plan guiding the building of this Institute was to regard psychiatry as the keystone of the whole arch of sciences. Now psychology alone and by itself is inadequate; it needs the support and auxiliary work of other sciences. The psychological group of sciences is to furnish the guiding principle of abnormal mental life-history, a principle that should control and at the same time be verified by the researches of the medico-biological group of sciences. Given some key to the general *modus operandi* by psychological investigation of some very carefully selected psychopathological case, a case furnishing crucial tests, the work of the medico-biological group of the sciences becomes subject to control. We know where to direct it. We are then under the guidance of a general hypothesis of the phenomena of insanity, know what facts to *select* from the work of the medico-biological group and how to *use* them. It is only under such conditions that we are enabled to *make pathological anatomy of great value, because we can interpret its results in relation to the living phenomena*, and it is only under such conditions that pathological anatomy will cease to be a dead science and will become a really living science. Most assuredly, then, to find some foundation for psychiatric research, we must begin at the living phenomena, find some key to their nature, and then only test and verify this theory by anatomy, chemistry and other sciences.

One can perceive that *the mainstay of this Institute is the field of the psychiatrist himself;* only we feel sure that at first we must begin in the investigation of abnormal mental phenomena outside of the hospital where they are less complicated. After some general key is found to explain these phenomena, the investigation may be extended little by little into the hospitals.

One point should be made quite distinct. *The plan and the motive inspiring the institution did not simply consist in assembling the various scientific departments under a common roof and bidding them work at the dead bodies of the insane.* Most assuredly not. This does not mean mutual co-operation of these sciences for the purpose of explaining the successions of the phenomena in abnormal mental life. The simple establishment of these departments in a common home does not mean *correlation* of the work toward a definite aim. All these departments might be established and although doing "work," giving forth "results," and industriously stimulating the same kind of activity in the hospitals, might leave us in the end not one whit nearer the laws and principles of abnormal phenomena of consciousness.

One might even add psychology to this group of sciences, and if one chooses the kind of scholastic "laboratory psychology" which is limited to the collection of statistical data of normal mental phenomena, such as reaction-time and the like, without in the least making a single step in advance. For the psychologist like other scientists falls into the notion that one is to be satisfied with collecting and cataloguing facts and data. Thus we find that some psychologists while piling up many data concerning the psychophysics of sensation and perception, forget to make use of the facts or to work out theories to correlate the facts. Their work bears an analogous relation to the true aim of psychology as that of the histologist or patho-anatomist to the science of function. The pathological anatomist piles up facts of abnormal structure as though they were explanations of abnormal function, whereas only through the study of the latter can he expect to gain an explanation of his facts, and a guide to discriminate the non-essential from the essential in his particular study.

Normal psychology must speculate as well as observe, and to speculate safely it must study the abnormal. If a department along the lines of simple "laboratory" psychology be added to the previous medico-biological group, the plan for psychiatric research would seem quite perfect. The delusion would indeed be quite strong. Psychology would then be working with the medico-biological group. The only trouble is that a psychology of numbers and incoherent "facts" by merely recording data and measurements can hardly give us a clew to the explanation of abnormal mental life. Collections of reaction-times among the insane and voluminous records of psychophysical measurements do not explain the abnormal phenomena of consciousness. Such a plan, even with the experimental type of psychological research included, might remain a *collection* but not an *organized correlation* of sciences in psychiatric research. Such a type of psychological research cannot possibly guide the work of the other sciences and the whole institution would fall short of its avowed purpose—the formulation of laws and principles of the phenomena of insanity.

In the amount of "work" related to insanity, however, that might be brought out of such an institution, its ultimate aim of explaining the living phenomena in insanity might be lost track of for some time. The example of such an institution would be pernicious. It would encourage others to fall into routine work and strongly discourage and delay the attempt to lead psychiatric research from the dominance of fact-collecting into the channel of the higher aim of elaborating the laws of mental life. The key to the finding of these laws lies in the domain of abnormal consciousness, not that the phenomena are at all different from the normal, but they better exhibit the phenomena of progressive dissociation. This furnishes the key.

I have desired to avoid turning psychiatric research into a cataloguing of facts in this institution, either under the guidance of pathological anatomy or of "laboratory psychology." On the grounds of expediency, however, it often seemed almost compulsory, from the pressure of bringing forth immediate results under the dominance of the mistaken medical idea of psychiatric research, to postpone the fulfillment of the ideal of this Institute and give over its energies to pathological anatomy and describe ganglion cell lesions wherever they could be found in the asylum mortuary and report it in the journals. The clinical histories could be written side by side with the morphological account, the interrelation of the two, the vital problem could be left for someone else to work out. I think, though, to relinquish the chosen aim of the research, even temporarily, for the sake of satisfying this mistaken notion for results, would have been dangerous. Had we started in this fashion, even holding in mind the ultimate aim of finding some working hypothesis of insanity to guide observation, it is quite likely that this aim would have been indefinitely postponed, and that we could have hardly paused long enough to work out the true aim of our endeavor. For the research is not isolated in this Institute; it extends out into twelve great hospitals with some twenty thousand patients and among one hundred to one hundred and twenty of our colleagues forming the staffs of these hospitals. It may be seen that the extent of the work of this Institute is rather extensive. I think it would be wrong to start right off simultaneously throughout these hospitals and deflect the work blindly into the channel of pathological anatomy and stop at the recording of the facts or with deductions so narrow as to be useless. It would be an unworthy response to so great an opportunity.

All over the civilized globe laboratory workers seem most actively engaged in recording observations gained by the Nissl method, although a good part of this activity seems to be conducted at the expense of reflections on the meaning of the observations. Such work by no means constitutes the central inspiration and motive of an institution for psychiatric research. We have to find a guide for this work and make it subserve some purpose in explaining the phenomena of insanity, or to show how these changes are effects of the morbid process concomitant with abnormal mental life. Work of this kind, and everything else, must not interfere with the proper aim of such an institution.

Although two years is an exceedingly short space of time, a wide range of cytological investigation of the neuron has been conducted more or less successfully. This morphological work embraces studies in the histogenesis of the neuron, in its comparative cytology through quite a number of invertebrates and lower vertebrates, and in many and varied pathological conditions in man, also experimentally induced in animals. All this work was not rushed into print as a mass of facts under the delusion that it explains the phenomena of insanity. These observations have, in the first place, been *used* for the formation of a general theory of the phenomena of insanity, and, secondly, *they have been used to lend support to the theory of neuron energy*, and, finally, the facts have been used to explain, as it seems to us, the mechanism of certain phases of mental and nervous disease process. Thus an explanation was found of peripheral neuritis, tabes, general paresis, and of a large part of the system diseases of the spinal cord and brain, such as combined sclerosis, amyotrophic lateral sclerosis, Landry's paralysis, pernicious anæmia, sclerosis, and of a large part of the whole problem of fibre death in the nervous system. *This has been accomplished by working out the significance of the migration of the neuron nucleus and the excretion of the metaplasm particles.**

Chapter XVIII.

MEDICINE AND PSYCHIATRY.

I have spoken somewhat freely of the pressure for results and its bad influence on the growth of a young institution, with the risk of having it fall amiss all around, both to the physician and the psychiatrist. If it concerned this Institute only it would certainly not be said, it would be a most unhappy return for the magnificent opportunity granted us by the directors of the hospitals and our Commission in Lunacy. If, however, this pressure for premature results is liable to depress and pervert

* An account of this work will appear in a future number of the Archives of Neurology and Psychopathology.

the progress of the science of psychiatry in general, it becomes a very serious matter and demands consideration.

In medicine there are an enormous number of eager, active "workers" in hundreds of laboratories vying with each other in the accomplishment of mechanical desk work on dead tissues. Every university has them—their name is legion. A new dye, a new technical method is a boon to them, it opens a new field for more "work." The cause of the phenomena is neglected, the process of transition of cause into effect dwindles out of sight. By its very volume and momentum, by the force of example, the influence of all this laboratory "work" widens and deepens the stress to conform to it.

The principal cause of this unintelligent vain labor and travail is our unfortunate manner of medical education. It is the fault of those who teach medicine. We fail to give our students so much as an inkling into the philosophy of medicine; we lead them to believe that the great goal of good work is the noting down of details. Observation of details is indeed necessary, but reflection and the use of the methods of seeking after causes are as much requisite, and possibly far more indispensable. The result is that too many men leave the medical university without knowing what science really means. They are possessed of the idea that science consists solely in observation of desultory facts and in aimless experimentation, and they consequently avoid the philosophy of science like a pest. They become ingrained with that false and mischievous notion that success is best achieved by sticking to one thing, one highly particularized line of observation.

The natural result of this training is that when men leave college and wish to enter the science of medicine, they go where desultory observation of new things has the greatest opportunity—pathological anatomy and bacteriology. They become skilful with technical methods and labor with the sense organs at laboratory desks despising all mental activity. The banishment of reflection is with them the *sine qua non* of good scientific work. To make an attempt to understand the phenomena and form a hypothesis, then verify it and arrive at a theory is a sacrilege. Reflection is theorizing, metaphysics, or as some of the profession like to express themselves strongly in popular parlance, mere rot. Their conception of the aim of science would have been pitiable, had it not been so ludicrous; science, according to them, is a kind of dime museum where all sorts of odd things and new curiosities are to be collected for exhibition.

It would be absurd to think for a moment that facts are of no value in science—science must have facts, but they are relatively useless until we can give them a valuation by the methods of reasoning. Without training in the general principles of biology, general physiology and psychology, we can hardly expect the medical student to find the basis for any broad elaboration of facts. Many brilliant minds in this field do not lead their energies toward the higher motives of science, because of their training in medicine and the lack of correlation with other sciences. Thus, year by year, the army of "workers" grows and the influence of joining it becomes stronger by mere force of social suggestion and imitation. Let a man leave the work desk in the laboratory to reflect on a purpose for his work, to subordinate the aimless observation, mechanical experimentation to an idea, to formulate a problem, and straightway he is a deserter from the ranks and is branded as an "ideal" idler, as a metaphysician. So great is the conceit of these "workers," so narrow is their mental horizon that outside their field of occupation everything is regarded with an air of superiority and utter contempt. Thus to one of this type of "workers" a book was shown in manuscript form. He looked at it with great arrogance and asked: Anything about the Nissl stain? No. Then it must be metaphysics. When Egypt was conquered by the barbaric Arabs the problem was what to do with the great Alexandrian library. Is the Koran in it? the barbarian asked. No. Is it in the Koran? No. Then it is useless stuff; burn it! I do not know whether the laboratory patho-anatomists are direct descendants of those barbarians, but they are certainly their successors in spirit.

Another spur to the haste to record desultory scrappy descriptions of facts is the great number of journals in medicine. In medical science there must be at least six or seven hundred journals. This is about five times as many as any other science uses, and about five times as many as necessary for well considered, deliberate and valuable scientific contributions. The rest are too much in the nature of catalogues, and to search through them to find the occasional papers of value is indeed a task. The evil is happily overcome by the year books; although one often hears the exceedingly valuable work of those who cast out the chaff in the year books pitied by the "workers" as compilers. I think the service rendered to science by those who assemble these disjointed fragmentary descriptions in some succession and order, is as valuable, if not more so, than many of the contributions from the "workers."

Such unnecessary journals play no inconsiderable share in urging medical men to forget the true aim of science in the blind, feverish race for "facts." Every centre of research, every laboratory, seems to desire to individualize its work in a new journal. Before long it is quite liable to happen that the work has to be made to order to keep the journal going. The work has to be ground out on time. This is simply ruinous to the higher motive of science. One should think twice before starting a new medical journal, that is, if it purports to advance the science of medicine. If a journal is inaugurated, it is well to show its purpose, as Roux has done in the fine introduction to his journal.

It is unnecessary to allude to the similar baleful influence exerted by superfluous medical societies in spurring medical men along hasty mechanical lines of work. The effect of it all, however, whether from one direction or another, is to drive medical research into a beaten track. Medicine, headed by pathological anatomy and bacteriology, is becoming too much a school of desultory facts. In America, we are trying to drive science along with the same haste that is characteristic of activity in other walks of life. No sooner is a scientific institution inaugurated than results are immediately demanded. The task of conforming to this demand has been particularly hard in this Institute, for it had no precedent to follow; it had to plan out all of the work on an entirely new basis. Haste is the bane of scientific *research*.

In the pressure to bring out work, problems whereby work can be guided intelligently, problems anticipating the *renaissance* of psychiatry as a science have to be ruthlessly cast aside. An institute devoted to the science of psychiatry is like an organism, it must grow and develop, it cannot become great by the irrational demand of the "workers" in medicine to make hasty "work."

Medical training thwarts all endeavors to find a pathway for the progress of the science of psychiatry. Investigations in psychiatry are to follow the pattern of medical laboratory work, and that unless indulged in it all research is deemed a failure. If we have come to such a pass, it is indeed time to declare openly that medicine is no guide for the student of psychiatry.

Neurologists, pathologists, histologists and all those high sounding "ologists" think that they can afford to disdain, deride and even to slander and defame the psychiatrist and his science. As a matter of fact the investigator of abnormal consciousness, with his broad view of life and science, has certainly a larger horizon and wider scope for scientific thought. It is high time that the psychiatrist should free himself from the incubi and succubi, the medical "ologists," that have weighed on him for so long a time. In the *art* of psychiatry medicine has been and still is a great mentor; in the *science* of psychiatry medicine can only lead astray.

CONTENTS OF PREVIOUS NUMBERS.

STATE HOSPITALS BULLETIN, VOL. II.

No. 4—October.

No. 3—July.

No. 2—April.

No. 1—January.

State Hospitals Bulletin, Vol. I.

No. 4—October.

No. 3—July.

No. 2—April.

No. 1—January.

www.ingramcontent.com/pod-product-compliance
Lightning Source LLC
Chambersburg PA
CBHW032141230426
43672CB00011B/2412
* 9 7 8 3 7 4 1 1 7 1 8 9 5 *